FREE TO BREASTFEED

Voices of Black Mothers

Jeanine Valrie Logan

&

Anayah Sangodele-Ayoka

Praeclarus Press, LLC
2504 Sweetgum Lane
Amarillo, Texas 79124 USA
806-367-9950
www.PraeclarusPress.com

All rights reserved. No part of this publication may be reproduced or transmitted in any form, or by any means, electronic or mechanical, including photocopy, recording, stored in a database, or any information storage, or put into a computer, without the prior written permission from the publisher.

DISCLAIMER
The information contained in this publication is advisory only and is not intended to replace sound clinical judgment or individualized patient care. The author disclaims all warranties, whether expressed or implied, including any warranty as the quality, accuracy, safety, or suitability of this information for any particular purpose.

ISBN: 978-1-939807-18-2

©2014 Jeanine Valrie Logan & Anayah Sangodele-Ayoka. All rights reserved.

Cover Design: Cornelia Georgiana Murariu
Acquisition & Development: Kathleen Kendall-Tackett
Copy Editing: Judy Torgus and Katherine Barber
Layout & Design: Cornelia Georgiana Murariu
Operations: Scott Sherwood

Table of Contents

Foreword	5
Preface	9
How to Use this book	16
Chapter 1: This Legacy Is Rich—and It's Ours	19
Chapter 2: Myths & Barriers	39
Chapter 3: Healthy Mama, Thriving Baby	59
Chapter 4: When the Bough Breaks	77
Chapter 5: Breastfeeding Warriors	99
Chapter 6: Coming to an End	133
Useful Terms	145
Resources	153
Contributors	157

Foreword

I got pregnant while training with women's national volleyball team. Breastfeeding was far away from my mind since I had, like, negative-A cups! But once the initial shock of the pregnancy set in, I began to romanticize what it would be like to hold, cuddle, and even nurse a baby.

I knew that I wanted to breastfeed because both my mother and sister did, and they were both there to share their experiences and support. The image that was impressed upon my mind was me looking down at my newborn son suckling gently while I stroked his soft hair, and feeling the pure joy and accomplishment that I was the only one to give him the nourishment he demanded. *That was just a dream!*

My son and I struggled at the beginning because he had a very shallow latch, and every time he latched on it was extremely painful. Fortunately, I had my mother there in the first few weeks to encourage me and reassure me that he would pick it up, and to give him time to learn to open his mouth. I also had a strong let-down that was causing him to choke when he latched on. I called the local *La Leche League* chapter to help me, and they explained to me the built-in supply and demand that our breasts have, and that it would balance out on its own. In my sleep-deprived state, I did not want to hear that; I needed a quick fix to get my baby fed so I could get some rest.

My husband was very supportive of me breastfeeding, and understood how important it was for both me and the baby, so he would take the baby at night, and I would get some much-needed rest. But right around three weeks we started hitting our groove, and I finally felt the joy and accomplishment that I dreamed about. I took great pride in knowing that I was built to provide the exact nourishment that my baby needed, that no one else could give him what he needed but me.

Even though I struggled at the beginning and needed the encouragement and support from my mother, husband, and the larger breastfeeding communities. I also drew upon my time with the U.S. Women's National Volleyball Team. During the first year of the four-year training block, our head coach called us all into his office and asked us if we could handle working as hard as we possibly could for four years to become Olympians. And at the end, not making it. I originally thought I could not handle it for fear of failure. I had never failed at anything. When it came to sports especially—I always succeeded, so the very thought of not being picked and obtaining my goal was very scary.

Over the next few years, fear engulfed me because I thought I might not make it. After childbirth, I found myself slipping into a similar space when I was struggling with my son's latch in the early weeks. But I did not let the fear overcome me! I had the resolve to say, *"I am going to give breastfeeding everything that I have because it's not only about me, but the foundation for my son's health depends on me seeing through my pain."*

I did not make the 2012 Olympics, but I learned that I have a choice to choose joy and enjoy the process over being fearful. I will admit that I didn't enjoy the entire process of breastfeeding, but I was able to snap out of my mini-setbacks and see the bigger picture quicker than before. I feel pure joy when I look into my now 14-month-old son's eyes and stroke his soft curls. He suckles just as gently as I originally imagined. It didn't happen on my time, but it happened and that's all that matters.

For me, breastfeeding is the ultimate way for you to connect with your baby. My milk is more than just nourishment for Judah. When he's scared, anxious, or just wants some cuddles, he knows where to turn. And the icing on the cake is that my body benefits from him nursing since I'm constantly burning calories. Baby weight?!? I think not! The benefits of breastfeeding far outweigh the minor struggles, and I believe that more Black women would breastfeed if they were exposed to more positive stories. It's vital that Black women know that they are equipped with everything they need physically to breastfeed, and that there are awesome outlets—like this book—to get emotional support.

The more Black women that are talking about breastfeeding—or even just nursing in a Starbucks—allows for breastfeeding to become natural and no longer taboo in our culture. I commend every mother that attempts to breastfeed her baby, whether it is one week or two years, you are amazing and more powerful than you will ever know.

Angie Forsett,
Three-time All-American in Volleyball, member, U.S. National Team

Preface

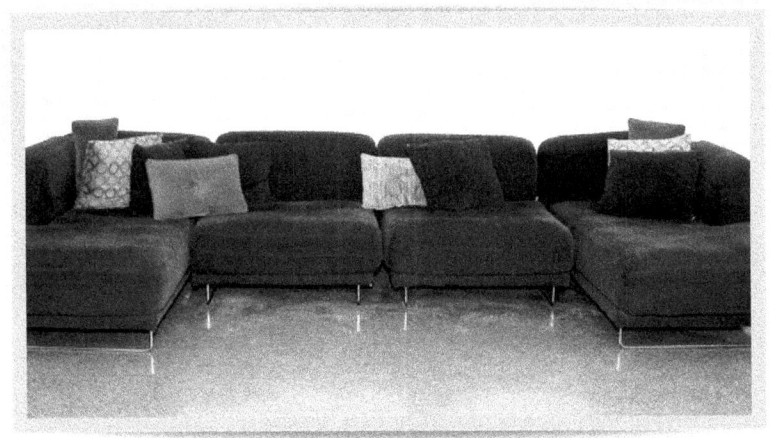

Anayah Sangodele-Ayoka

We may be very well living in the age of too much information. At the swipe of a fingertip and blink of an eye, we have access to text, video, and sounds from the furthest reaches of the planet—even universe. Our only limitations may be what we have the audacity to seek. Or maybe, it's preparation.

You see, despite having all this access to information and advice, we still find ourselves in a battle of David and Goliath proportions to make most African-American women aware of the great benefits of mother's milk and breastfeeding. Even greater is the battle to ensure societal support. For African-American women, babies, and families, this is of special significance.

Let us contrast the rates of childhood obesity, asthma, and breast cancer we face with the reality that each of these is specifically known to be decreased with exclusive breastfeeding.

The constituents of breast milk are specially crafted to meet the child's needs at each stage of her development. And while developing the maternal-child bond on this side of pregnancy involves many components, doing so through breastfeeding is literally a treasure trove.

Personally, I had little to no anxiety about being pregnant or even giving birth. However, anyone who knew me at the time would get an earful about how unprepared I felt for actually being a mother. I worried about making the wrong decision to set my child on a poorly fated life course.

Perhaps this is the perpetual anxiety of all parents. About 45 minutes after being born, Sangojobi and I lay in bed with him latched to my breast and those anxieties were changed.

Through our 22-month (and counting) journey of breastfeeding, we both had a safe haven. Even through our most challenging moments, that moment of pause has been the catalyst for me embracing motherhood as an empowered woman.

My child and I learned each other's facial expressions, moods, and rhythms. I have literally been his food, comfort, and medicine, as if this mother's milk was nature's own way of showing me that I had everything I needed to mother.

When we began the Brown Mamas Breastfeed Project, we felt the audacious responsibility of increasing the visibility of Black mothers who breastfeed.

I never considered not breastfeeding because I had seen my mother, her friends, and my own friends do it. I was a breastfed child and knew where to turn for support if I found difficulty.

For the vast majority of us, this is not the case. For this reason, we are extremely grateful for these celebrity mothers (and mothers of would-be celebrities) for letting the world know that they are Free to Breastfeed too.

- *Erykah Badu, singer/songwriter*
- *Beyonce Knowles, singer*
- *Ananda Lewis, TV personality*

- *Michelle Obama, lawyer and First Lady of the United States*
- *Deloris Jordan, author and mother of athlete Michael Jordan*
- *Jada Pinkett-Smith, actress and author*
- *Mariah Carey, singer*
- *Laila Ali, boxer*
- *Tia Mowry-Hardict, actress*
- *Essence Atkins, actress*
- *Jourdan Dunn, model*
- *Christina Milian, pop star*
- *Kimora Lee, model and entrepreneur*
- *Candace Parker, WNBA player*
- *Celest Arantes do Nascimento, mother of athlete Edson "Pelé" Arantes do Nascimento*
- *Brynn Cameron, WNBA player*
- *Lisa Leslie, WNBA player*
- *Sheryl Swoopes, WNBA player*
- *Halle Berry, actress*
- *Lisa Bonet, actress and mother of model, Zoe Kravitz*
- *Solange Knowles, singer/songwriter and model*
- *Amel Larrieux, singer/songwriter*

With these women, and the brave mothers who shared their private stories in the pages to follow, we're in good company.

Anayah Sangodele-Ayoka

Jeanine Valrie Logan

Growing up, I don't recall witnessing any of my family members pregnant, let alone breastfeeding. I never saw it. Conversations I had with my mother about her own breastfeeding experience were short and to the point. You see, my mother did not breastfeed me. Being poor and young, and having had a medically managed caesarean birth, she was dissuaded from breastfeeding. At the time, the doctor's reasoning seemed valid: my mother began having cystic lumps removed from her breast at age 13.

At 23, and a new mother, she was told by her doctors that if she breastfed it would increase her chances of getting breast cancer. What we know now is that breastfeeding actually not only reduces one's risk for developing breast cancer, but risk is also exponentially reduced the longer one breastfeeds. This information is major for Black women who die from breast cancer at a rate four times greater than White women.

When talking about her missed opportunity to breastfeed, the regret and sadness in my mother's voice always shook me. It wasn't until much later, until I understood the gloriousness of breastfeeding that I recognized what she may have felt.

My mother died February 11, 1998 from metastatic breast cancer, almost four years to the date of her diagnosis. She was 43 years old. My sickly childhood, and my mother's illness and eventual death, all played a role in how I came to breastfeeding activism; with arms wide open and a hungry commitment to breastfeeding my own child(ren). *But this is my history.*

Preface

In conceptualizing this book and the misconception behind the belief that Black women don't breastfeed, I was truly interested in hearing about how other Black women came to join this breastfeeding journey. My mother's voice and memories were a constant presence enveloping me throughout the process of this book. Much of this book was edited in the wee hours of the morning; sometimes while nursing my own 18-month-old daughter, Ahimsa.

These stories and the stories of other Black breastfeeding mothers, motivated me and nourished my spirit with every page turn. Often times I found myself screaming out, crying from the sheer beauty of the sacred memories shared, laughing loudly, or sighing out loud in solidarity from tales of pain, poor latch, healing, and perseverance.

Although we are overly excited about what we are about to share with you, we know that this collection of stories is not complete. There are millions of stories we do not share; experiences of Black teen mothers, Black queer mothers, Black adoptive mothers, Black mothers who are within the prison industrial complex; the list can go on and on. Knowing this, we hope that these stories will act as a starting point for discussions within our communities, a steadfast support in those difficult moments, and a self-empowering guide when discussing one's breastfeeding goals with family, friends, partners, and health care providers.

Because breastfeeding IS the revolution...
Jeanine Valrie Logan

How to Use this Book

Within these pages are the tender inner thoughts of African-American women, with narratives, until now, unpublished. Each chapter covers a new and engaging theme as it is our intention for readers to be able to enjoy this book in a nonlinear fashion.

- In *Chapter 1,* we hear from mothers reflecting on breastfeeding as a legacy that they are either initiating in their sphere of influence, or picking up from women before them.

- *Chapter 2* addresses the many myths and barriers women face to successful breastfeeding, from negative naysayers to misinformed health professionals. Unfortunately, the fact that breastfeeding passed out of the mainstream for over four decades has meant that many health professionals are uneducated about best practices. Every breastfeeding mother should know that painful, chafed, or bleeding nipples are not normal, but can probably be overcome with the informed support of knowledgable peer supporters and lactation consultants.

- In *Chapter 3,* we get a unique glimpse into the interconnectedness of mother and baby's physical and emotional health.

- In *Chapter 4,* mothers share surprising tips they've used to troubleshoot discomfort or circumstances that might have compromised their breastfeeding relationship.

- *Chapter 5* picks up on the thread of empowerment with reflections from mothers who have gone above and beyond to nurse multiple children, sometimes simultaneously, and sometimes not their own.

🐦 The reflections in *Chapter 6* remind us that even this relationship must end for the baby to blossom. These pieces are heartfelt, and if you're anything like us, you should have tissues close at hand.

Throughout this book there will be terms that you may not be familiar with. You will find a *glossary* of these helpful terms following Chapter 6.

We have also provided a list of books, websites, and videos that we believe are relevant to Black breastfeeding women in the *Resources* section.

Lastly, you can learn more about the writers of these honest and powerful reflections in the *Contributors'* section.

Enjoy!
Free to Breastfeed

Chapter 1

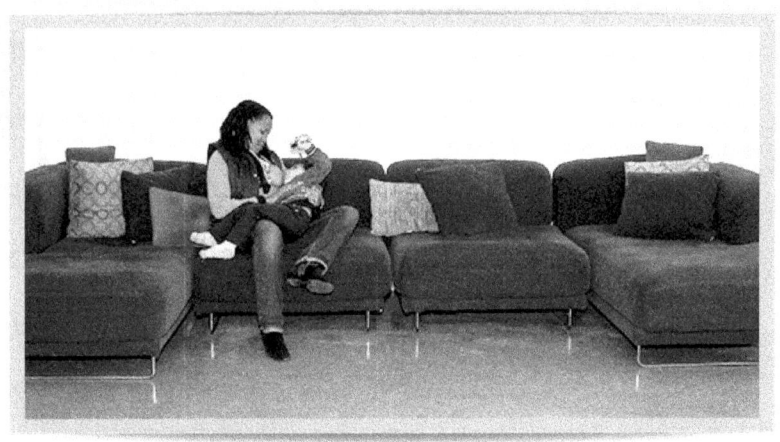

This Legacy Is Rich—and It's Ours

Whether they approached their breastfeeding journey by reading lots of books, or by heeding the whispers of intuition, these women's stories are a testament. These are the reflections of women proud to have shared their mother's milk in the tradition of countless women before them.

Chapter 1: This Legacy Is Rich—and It's Ours

In 2011, we hosted an online viral project called the *Brown Mamas Breastfeed Project,* where we asked Black women to share pictures of themselves breastfeeding.

This was one of those humbling submissions.

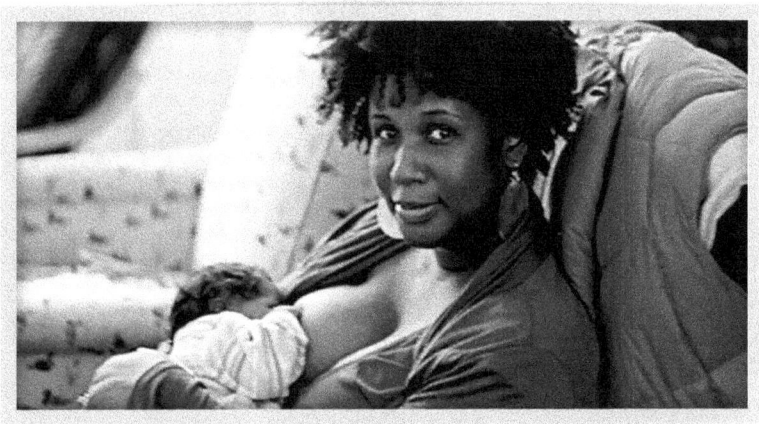

Brown Mamas Breastfeed
Dee and Wren

My three older kids breastfed for almost 2 years, 2 1/2 years, and 3 1/2 years, respectively. It seemed like the easiest choice. Wren has been nursing for 16 months.

My family members all breastfed and I always knew I would, too. I love the special connection to my little one and being forced to slow down and enjoy the pace of mothering a young child.

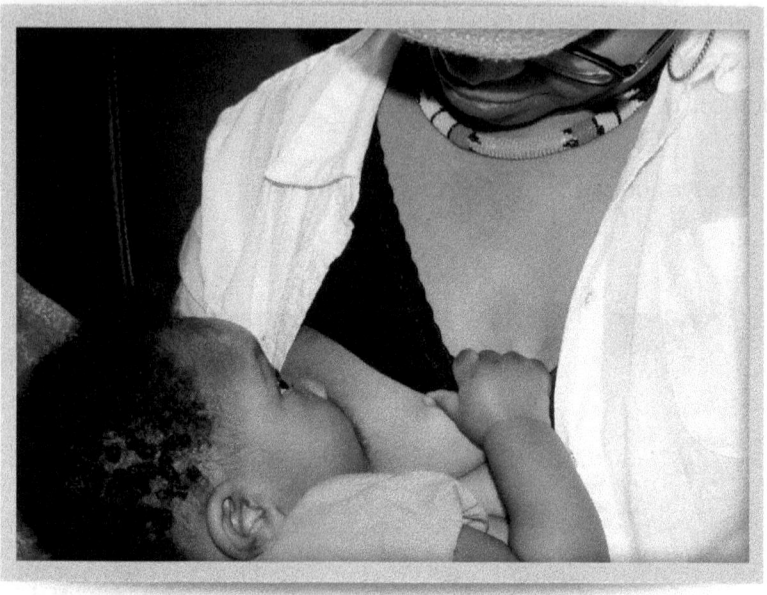

Ode to Fenugreek
by Jackie Joice

I come from a long line of non-breastfeeding (or breastfed) women. I wasn't breastfed, my mother wasn't breastfed, nor did she breastfeed my siblings, and as far as I know, my grandmother wasn't breastfed either. So naturally, I'd have some reservations about breastfeeding. Statistically, African-American women represent the ethnic group least likely to breastfeed, and if they do breastfeed it's only for a short duration of time.

Today, breastfeeding advocates and organizations seem to be doing more to reach the African-American community. In my case, I was torn about nursing, I thought it would be inconvenient, painful, and difficult. I couldn't imagine a little human being

Chapter 1: This Legacy Is Rich—and It's Ours

sucking on my breast. One woman that I met at a Ladyfest music festival, in what is referred to as the Inland Empire of Southern California, described her experience to me regarding breastfeeding and said, *"It felt like shards of glass flowing through my mammary glands."* Really? *"Shards of glass?"* Oh I can't wait to experience this sensation!

After hearing that woman's harrowing story, I was absolutely terrified. My husband stated that he would support my decision either way. However, his views on breastfeeding were completely different from mine. He was breastfed and came from a culture (Ghana, West Africa) that considered breastfeeding second nature.

In fact, when I visited Ghana in 2002, I often saw women breastfeeding infants that weren't biologically their own. Oh, the horror! Had I known then what I know now about breast milk and breastfeeding, my opinion would have been quite different.

I became pregnant in 2009. It wasn't until my belly was the first thing anyone saw coming around the corner that my views about breastfeeding changed. The experience of my daughter moving and responding to our voices inside my womb was life-changing and affirming.

At the same time, a very good friend of mine, Tanya, from Poughkeepsie, NY, mailed me a package with all types of literature on breastfeeding. She runs her own business, one in which she makes natural cloth menstrual pads, postpartum and nursing pads. She asked me what my favorite colors were and made me a whole bunch of custom designed nursing pads.

During my 39th week, I had to have a c-section. I had no idea that the c-section would interrupt my hormonal process of lactation causing my breast milk not to flow right away. While I was hospitalized and recovering, I began breastfeeding my daughter with colostrum. I wasn't positioning my daughter correctly, so within a day or so, my breasts were sore and my nipples were cracked and bleeding, especially on my left side. Yikes!

Remember those shards of glass? My fears had actualized. I was so distraught because my daughter would go into these ravenous fits, like in the movie, *The Exorcist,* because she was hungry.

We began to supplement with formula until the pain subsided, and I was able to spend some time with a lactation consultant. The lactation consultant showed me how to position my daughter so that she would "latch on" correctly. I was willing to keep trying, although the pain was unbearable.

Once I was released from the hospital, I decided to do some research regarding my delayed milk supply. I consider myself a pretty informed herbalist, however, I didn't know off hand which herbs served as galactagogues.

A galactagogue is a substance that induces lactation. I knew which herbs toned the uterus (red raspberry being a favorite), and conditioned the reproductive system, like red clover, but I had no idea which ones increased milk supply. I discovered that fennel and fenugreek were two seeds that increased the milk supply. I had some fennel on hand, but discovered it was too strong a diuretic for me. However, the golden seed fenugreek was my remedy.

Chapter 1: This Legacy Is Rich—and It's Ours

Fenugreek (Latin name, *Trigonella foenum-graecum*) is of the pea family *(Fabaceae)*. Fenugreek has several medicinal and culinary uses; like flavoring for imitation maple syrup. Speaking of maple syrup, one of the side effects of consuming fenugreek tea is that it seeps from your pores. In other words, the perspiration from your breast area will smell like maple syrup. Your infant's poop will be scented too. Fenugreek also affects your blood sugar levels, so before trying any herbal remedies, please check with your physician first.

I knew of an Indian spice store in Little India that had been in business for years. We decided to drive there and buy the seeds in bulk.

The aroma in the store was a mixture of curry, turmeric, and other Indian and Mediterranean spices. There were huge burlap sacks of spices and seeds located in the back room. An elderly Indian man paid me no mind as I observed him scooping loose spices and seeds and packaging them.

We patrolled the aisles of various culinary condiments and seasonings as Indian music played in the background. Suddenly, as we turned yet another corner in the cramped store, there was a glare of golden light that gleamed from one particular aisle. We soon discovered it was the auspicious fenugreek seed on the shelf in multiple sizes of bags. The shelves glowed with this magical seed. It was very inexpensive, too.

As soon as I arrived home, I boiled a tablespoon of fenugreek seeds in about two cups of water until the water turned golden.

I drank about two cups per day. The results were impressive. My breast milk increased almost overnight, and now I was a human dairy queen. By the way, no one informed me about what would happen once my breasts became engorged. One day, as I nursed Sunshine, one of my breasts sprung a leak! EEEEP! It was quite funny, to be honest.

Once my breast milk was regularly flowing I became real confident. I even went out and purchased a breast pump.

After I got the hang of using the breast pump, I stored bags and bags of my breast milk in the freezer. I did some self-portraits of my daughter on my breast for a brochure contest on *Breastfeeding Awareness*.

In conclusion, I hope that my story encourages women—especially African-American women—to breastfeed their babies as long as they can. If a mother cannot breastfeed, she can at least use a breast pump. The important thing is that the infant consumes breast milk as long as possible. Now of course, there are a few medical reasons why some women cannot breastfeed.

I also understand that it is a personal choice, and no woman should feel guilty for choosing not to breastfeed. There are plenty of man-made formulas that are recommended by doctors that may provide some of the same benefits, but of course not nearly all of the benefits of breast milk. Hopefully women, and especially African-American women, will take into consideration the multiple psychological (bonding), and nutritional benefits that a baby receives from nursing.

Besides, nursing has many benefits to the mother as well, like reducing the risk of breast cancer, and burning up to 500 calories a day! And lastly, if your breast milk production is low, do not fret; there's always the golden, magical fenugreek seed to assist you.

There's Life in Them There Hills
by Stacey Gibson

"I had milk," she said. "I was pregnant with Denver, but I had milk for my baby girl. I hadn't stopped nursing her when I sent her on ahead. All I knew was I had to get my milk to my baby girl. Nobody was going to nurse her like me...nobody had her milk but me. I told [the women on the wagon] to put sugar water in cloth to suck from so when I got there in a few days she wouldn't have forgot me. The milk would be there and I would be there with it."

Toni Morrison, Beloved

I remember first encountering this passage in Toni Morrison's crushing book, *Beloved,* and feeling the weight of the words. I was not entirely certain of all the implications and complexity of the lines, but I knew truthtelling when I saw it. Sure, I could merge the letters to form the words to read the sentence, but the depth of the meaning took years to take root, blossom, and then cultivate.

To know that the main character of that book, Sethe, suffered the turmoil of being gang raped while six months pregnant, and bearing a freshly shredded, open-fleshed back wound, with feet so swollen she was only able to crawl through the hungry back hills of Kentucky; all because she knew she had the milk her older daughter needed. Her moving words were: *"All I knew was I had to get my milk to my baby girl"* (Morrison, p. 17).[1]

Black women have never had the luxury of the wet nurse, or the callous aloofness that was often attributed to white women, because they were relieved that someone else (a Black woman)

---

1) Toni Morrison, *Beloved* (New York: Alfred A Knopf 1987), 17

would totally and completely care for their [white] child when they didn't feel like it. Very little was—or is— romantic about being *"the help."*

Black diasporic women always knew that in handing off burdens to someone *"beneath"* us, there was, and still is, and no one we trust who will work unwaveringly to pick up, carry, and take care of our responsibilities. Sister Zora Neal Hurston shared that insight matter-of-factly in, *Their Eyes Were Watching God*.

During our most brutal oppression, we created systems that ensured our babies' survival, and that they made sure they had as much nourishment as possible, even though they could be sold away in the dark of night.

The plantations, whose main crops were breeding Black babies, were fully stocked with women whose *"job"* it was to nurse the infants. As much as we know about the women-mothers-aunties-tanties-and-ma'am's who threw away their babies, or chose infanticide rather than enslavement, there were many, many, many more women-mothers-aunties-tanties-and-ma'ams who took our great, great, great, great, great grandparents, and put that baby to her breast, only to later ask, *"Do this one have a name yet?"*

That milk coming from that "fictional character's" breasts, in those hungry hills of Kentucky, matters right now. Black women have always made do in the most dire and desperate of circumstances, and somehow managed to keep folk alive. They did so without maids, mint juleps, and the ever-so-convenient "break from it all."

I recently read an interview with folk singer and educator, Ella Jenkins, in a March 2011 issue of *Streetwise* magazine. In the interview, she talks about growing up poor in the city [Chicago], but always having food with sustenance and heartiness that was still nutritionally sound. I thought about this on a recent trip with a group of Black mothers and daughters, and was disheartened when the adult women (not the children), started chanting loudly "MIC-KEY-D's MIC-KEY-D's" at 9:45 p.m. even though dinner had been served at 5:30 p.m.

There are life-giving blueprints in the painful passages our foremothers went through. I understand that exposure to some of their pain will unfurl anguish so riotous it may break parts of ourselves we are afraid to explore.

Currently there are more choices for dangerous pseudo-foods, and less access to widespread sustainable systemic sustenance. Our relationship with nourishment—not just food—is one of our many disrupted pathways, and begs for our attention or we will pay with our death. Our children struggle to digest and absorb empty pseudo-foodstuffs as we struggle to maintain a manageable weight.

So to stand on the edge of a noisy cataclysmic world stage and watch large numbers of us struggle to consistently feed our own properly makes me wonder deeply about those women, like Sethe Suggs. Somehow they knew no matter how bastardized, distorted, and fractured their humanity was, moving that milk was a radical act of resistance where a Black woman took a stance and owned motherhood/mothering at a time when she was worth everything—and nothing—all at once.

These women knew how to navigate and set up systems to save what life they could. We must do the very same at this moment, especially because that milk coming from that *"fictional character's"* breasts, in those hungry hills of Kentucky, matters right now.

Nourishing My Babies, Myself
by Barbara Mhangami-Ruwende

As I lay on the operating table, I heard a deep gutsy cry from my 9 lb 10 oz baby girl. She had taken her time, coming into the world at 41 weeks, and after 18 hours of unproductive labor. My doctor performed a c-section, and as he placed Chichi on my chest, my heart lurched and I burst into tears. I fell in love and knew instinctively from that moment on my whole being was for her benefit.

After I was settled in my room, a nurse brought Chichi to me to breastfeed. I had been asked prior to my labor and delivery whether or not I intended to breastfeed. I found the question quite bizarre because I had never thought that breastfeeding was optional. This was the American way.

I come from Zimbabwe, where breastfeeding is the norm. From my experience, women who give formula do so as supplementation to the breast, and this is usually only done when the mother returns to work or has to be away from her baby for extended time periods.

However, for many women even supplementing is not an option because of the costly nature of baby formula and the fear of making the baby ill by using inadequately sterilized bottles or contaminated water. I was surprised when, as I held Chichi, hungrily taking in her every feature, a lactation specialist came into the room to "facilitate" the breastfeeding. After a few frustrating minutes with the specialist manhandling my breasts, pinching my nipple, and pushing the baby's head towards it, I politely told her to give the baby and me a few minutes alone to try to figure it out by ourselves.

Chapter 1: This Legacy Is Rich—and It's Ours

My great-grandmothers, grandmothers, aunts, and mother had all successfully nursed their babies without the assistance of any lactation specialist.

I knew that if I held my baby to the breast, she would open her mouth and latch on. I had seen this so many times in Zimbabwe: on buses, on park benches, in the market, at parties, and in doctors' waiting rooms. Breastfeeding is accepted as a part of the culture, and the breast of a nursing woman is not seen as a sex object, but as a source of sustenance. Strangers will offer a mother with a baby a seat on the bus so that she can feed her baby, or offer to carry her luggage so she can feed the baby.

The specialist came back into the room to find a tired but contented mother and child resting comfortably on the pillows. Chichi was getting nourishment and immunity from the colostrum in my breast, while I was getting spiritual sustenance, and the rush of oxytocin that would eventually restore my body and my uterus to its pre-pregnancy state.

I nursed Chichi for 18 months because we both enjoyed the closeness that this intimate time afforded us. I nursed in public, much to the horror of many people. However, I have never been one to care too much about the opinion of strangers, and this instance was no different. As long as I was not breaking any laws, and my baby was hungry, I would breastfeed her.

I greeted my second daughter, Kai, with a warm breast, and for 10 months of her life, she and I bonded during nursing time. She weaned herself after 10 months. Nursing her was a very different experience from nursing Chichi because they are different personalities. I got to know their individual quirks and reactions as infants just from tuning into them while they nursed at my breast. This knowledge was very useful because it informed my responses to each of them, and I could parent them by providing for their individual needs.

My twins, Shami and Tendo, were also breastfed, but the experience was very different from nursing my singletons. There were times when I would nurse them one at a time, and other moments when I would nurse the two of them together. I also had to pump a lot more than I did with the singletons in order to stimulate high milk production.

It was a very busy time for our family. However, I found one-on-one time with the twins during breastfeeding sessions. Although they are identical, I got to know each of them and to experience their unique characters.

As I reflect on the experience of breastfeeding my children, I recall cracked nipples, engorged breasts, and embarrassing leaks. Yet not once during that time did I consider formula feeding a viable option.

The knowledge that I was giving my children the best there possibly was in terms of infant nutrition was enough incentive to go through the rough patches.

The nipples healed, I pumped when the pressure became unbearable, and I used breast pads if I was going to be away from the babies for a long time. I had very good support in my husband and my mother, who would often feed the babies bottled breast milk so that I could have a break. Despite the moments of difficulty, the moments of pure joy and contentment were greater. The memories of quiet tenderness are more dominant than those of discomfort.

The period of breastfeeding was one of intense awareness for me. I was aware of how and what I ate because I knew this affected milk quality. I included lots of fruit, vegetables, whole grains, and high-quality protein sources into my diet, and avoided fatty, sugary, artificially flavored foods. I was acutely aware of any increase in stress levels because my milk output would decrease. I, therefore, made sure I got adequate sleep and exercise. I was relaxed, and avoided situations that were upsetting.

These healthy lifestyle habits were ones I would continue with long after I stopped breastfeeding. The result is that I lost all the weight inevitably gained during pregnancy, and I have four happy, healthy girls, aged 10, 8, and 5 years. I continue to take care of myself now, as I did when I was nursing, ensuring that I am giving my daughters the best of me now as I did when they were infants. *This makes me a very busy, but fulfilled mother.*

Let A Tradition Be Born
by Natalie D. Preston-Washington

There is no legacy of breastfeeding on my side of the family. I am my parent's only child and my mother did not breastfeed me. Nor did her sister breastfeed her daughter, which explains why my aunt was so curious and attentive when I would breastfeed in her presence.

Is he still sucking?
Does it hurt?
How long you gonna breastfeed?
Is he finished?

Every visit. Every nursing session. The same series of questions.

At first I was put off by her extreme curiosity. Then, after speaking with my mother and learning how breastfeeding was not embraced "back then," I understood. My aunt had not experienced it firsthand and there we were in living color for her to observe. From that point on I viewed her queries as an opportunity to enlighten.

Yes, he is still nursing. Sometimes he will break for a bit and then resume. At first it hurt when he latched on until we both figured out what we were doing. Now it's easy breezy...I committed to three months, then six months, now who knows? I am in no rush to give Luke milk from a cow or some artificial source. Yes, he is asleep. A successful nursing session!

I find it interesting that slaves nursed their children, and their master's kids. And, I would assume that women breastfed during the depression years, if for no other reason than financial motivation. However, my mom's civil rights generation appears to have dropped the baton during the sexy '70s, when I was born.

In 2011, visits to my OB/Gyn have not convinced me that breastfeeding is on a resurgence. I see a clear delineation between the nursers and the nots.

Families should be the first line of support when it comes to breastfeeding. If a mom is able to produce milk, then she should be educated, encouraged, and enabled with the necessary resources to breastfeed. The fact that milk is available from other non-maternal sources at little-to-no cost is irrelevant.

Likewise, as Black women who nurse, we should make it a point to educate, encourage, and enable other mothers to nurse. The fact that the other mothers are not relatives, or are of a different ethnicity, is irrelevant.

Woman to Woman
by Nilajah Brown

The first couple of days of nursing was nothing like I read in the books. My breasts became so engorged that my skin began to peel and my nipples were so raw. I had to walk around naked. I called my birth buddies and did everything they recommended...from taking a shower and letting the warm water sooth my breasts, to drinking herbal lactation-support concoctions.

After nothing worked, I sat quiet and that little voice (aka, my womanly intuition) told me to call my Auntie. Auntie said, *"Girl, tell that man to run get you some cabbage leaves and lay them on your breast."* I fell asleep with the leaves on my breast, and when I woke, my bed was soaked with milk. I was finally flowing again.

I now make sure I tell all the mamas I work with about the wonder of cabbage leaves. Some wisdom will never be found in books. It's just passed on from woman to woman.

Chapter 2

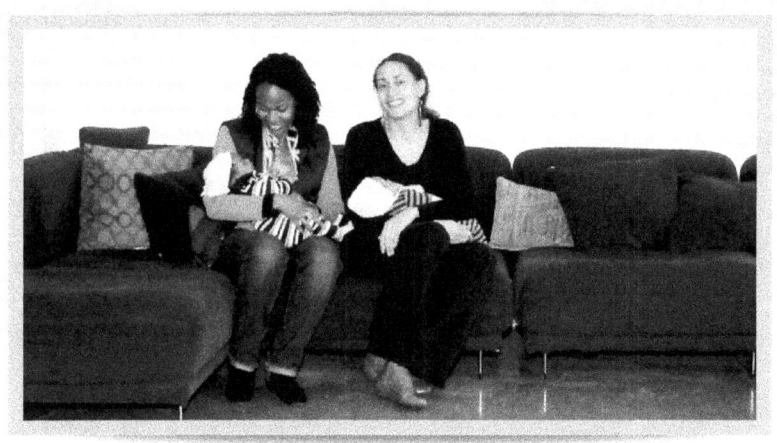

Myths and Barriers

They made this choice over and over again. These are the reflections of mothers who overcame obstacles and misinformation. Through their sacrifices, calls for support, withering resolve, and re-energized attempts, these women learned the ropes while climbing.

Chapter 2: Myths and Barriers

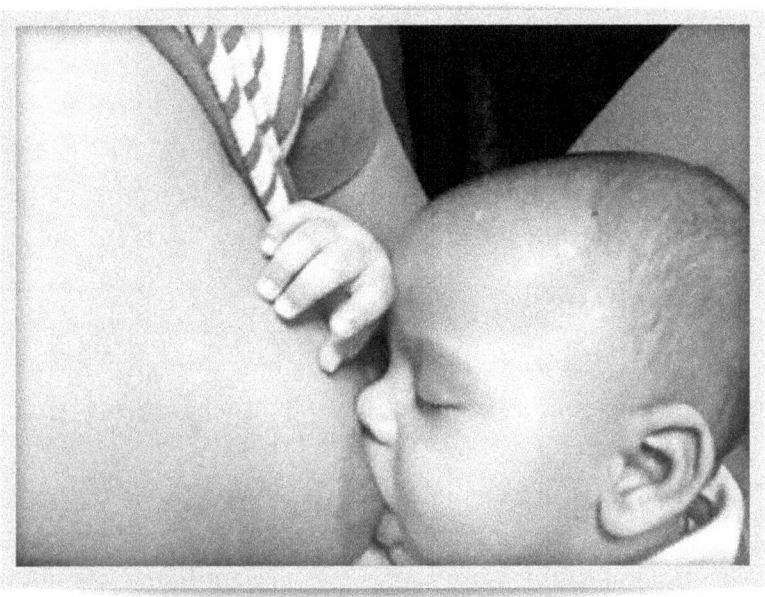

Beyond Words
by Sarah Beaty

Before I became a mother, breastfeeding was out of sight, out of mind. I really didn't have an opinion about it: good or bad. I didn't choose to breastfeed. Breastfeeding chose me. If that makes any sense at all.

When I looked at my firstborn laying on my chest, something clicked. The nurses cleaned her off and right away I said, *"When can I breastfeed her?"* They replied, *"Right now"* and she latched perfectly. Not everybody has a wonderful story like that, but the same thing happened with my son, Major. He latched perfectly, and we are still breastfeeding strong, and he is 8 months old.

One thing I did notice while at the hospital when my daughter Kiana was born, though, was that she kept throwing up.

The nurses told me that it was normal for babies to have a little reflux. I brought her home and she nursed great, but suffered from severe reflux. Spitting up out her nose, and choking on the spit up. This went on for a few weeks when I made up in my mind it must be my breast milk, and gave her some formula to see if she could handle it better. I was really confused thinking my milk was too thin. She wasn't gaining good weight and was really fussy.

At her first pediatric appointment at a month old, her doctor suggested adding rice cereal to her formula to thicken it, and told me she should hold her milk down better. I went from nursing exclusively to nursing 50% of the time, and the other 50% of the time giving her formula with rice cereal. Little did I know, that would be the beginning of the end of our breastfeeding relationship.

She still had severe acid reflux, so at her 2-month checkup, the doctor gave me a sample of Enfamil AR (formula specifically for babies with acid reflux) to see if that would help.

By then, my supply had diminished, and soon after that recommendation by my pediatrician she was fed Enfamil AR 100% of the time. The acid reflux still did not stop. So, at the 4-month checkup, the doctor put her on an acid reflux medicine. The combination of the medicine and Enfamil AR helped a lot. By the time she was 8 months old, she had completely stopped spitting up, and I started weaning her off the medicine. Looking back on the situation, if I had had the medical advice and support I needed, I would have nursed her well over 2 months.

My son, Major, has acid reflux now, and we are breastfeeding strong at 8 months old. He just started the acid reflux medicine a couple months ago and is doing great. We have no plans of stopping anytime soon.

My favorite thing about nursing is the convenience of night nursing. A combination of safe co-sleeping and night nursing allows me to get plenty of sleep. The piece of mind I have knowing that my baby is getting my milk, which is always sterile, is great too.

Also, I LOVE gazing in my baby's eyes. He then looks at me and we have a stare-down contest while he's nursing. Then he cracks a smile. It's special beyond words...

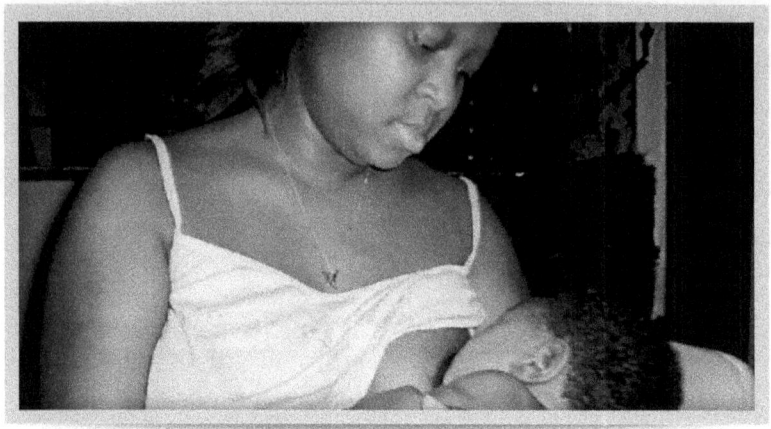

Free Food!
by Patrice London

I've exclusively breastfed my three daughters and plan to do the same with any other children I have in the future.

My first and second daughters self-weaned (due to birth control pills and the patch changing and depleting my milk supply) at around 18 months and 12 months.

When my youngest daughter arrived, I was using Natural Family Planning and because my milk wasn't affected, my daughter nursed until she was just three months away from her third birthday.

I'd always planned to nurse my children until at least 2 years of age, and was encouraged to do so by my husband's grandmother (who is from Guyana, South America). I believe that breastfeeding my children has greatly affected their overall health. They have no food allergies, and I can't say I remember the last time anyone has been sick. My youngest, who nursed the longest, has only had one fever and one cold in her life, and she is now 4 years old.

I am very proud of the fact that all of my children were breastfed, but I would never tell anyone it was easy. I have a cousin who breastfed her three girls quite easily with no problems at all, but that's not my story. I had cracked and bleeding nipples in the beginning with my first daughter because of inverted nipples, a poor latch, and virtually no help at all.

It was sheer determination that kept me going in spite of the pain and pitied looks from family, and horrific advice from my daughter's pediatrician, who advised me to supplement with formula for a week while the nipple that was worse off healed. I remember crying profusely, thinking I was killing my child when I learned that her weight had gone down after her birth, which no one bothered to tell me was completely normal.

We made it through in spite of it all. I threw out that formula before the week was over, and very shortly after, my first daughter had so many rolls, she was often referred to as the *"Michelin-man's baby"* or the *"bakery baby."*

When my second daughter came along five years later, I thought breastfeeding wouldn't be a problem since I knew what I was doing, and inverted nipples weren't an issue—but I was wrong. This baby didn't want to open her mouth wide enough, so again I had sore nipples. But this time I got help from my midwife, and that baby never had a drop of formula.

My third baby and I ended up in the office of a lactation consultant, and I felt like a complete moron having successfully breastfed two other children, but still having issues with the next. As horrible as things were at that time, it was short lived, and my youngest went on to breastfeed for the longest of all my girls so far.

I've never had any issues with breastfeeding in public, and could be found nursing my babies wherever we went including amusement parks, plays, restaurants, and even church. I even organized a Nurse-In at my local Applebee's in 2007 when there was a nationwide Nurse-In called by nursing mothers all over the U.S., when one woman in Kentucky was asked to leave Applebee's because she was making their other guests uncomfortable. It was a great experience that my two older daughters will always treasure.

As accustomed as I was to nursing my babies when they were younger, nursing a toddler was a very different experience. My oldest was a toddler when she stopped nursing (around 18 months), but my first and third daughters are very different people. My youngest liked to get into the oddest positions that often made me feel like we were a circus act, and she had this annoying habit of playing with the other nipple as she nursed on one breast.

I'd move her hand and try to occupy her, only to have that little hand creep right back to my free nipple (whether clothed or not), and start to twist, poke, and pull.

Nursing a toddler in public was very different too. I've never had anyone say anything to me, or even look at me funny, as most don't even know what I'm doing—they think I'm simply holding my baby—but I felt this self-imposed weird feeling about nursing my toddler in public. Of course the fact that she'd sometimes stand on my lap with her butt in the air nursing didn't help, but I quickly got over it.

I wish more Black women would breastfeed their babies full-term and not just a few weeks, months, or even just one year. The benefits are priceless, and like my husband says, *"it's FREE FOOD"!!*

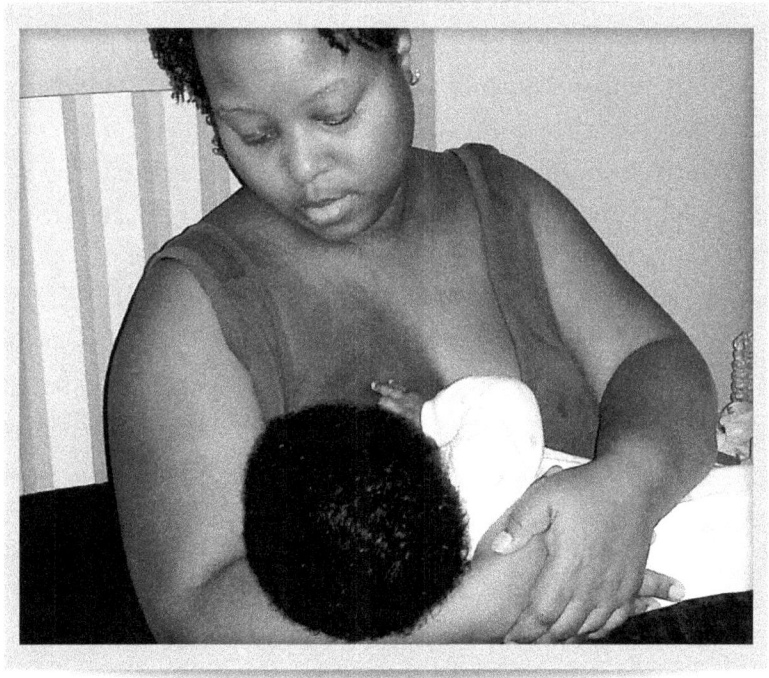

Retrograde Lullaby
by Mpho Venusmoon Majozi
(For Jabari)

Daily you give birth to me
What I conceive
Contacting in the wake
Of new vision
Pushed to gestate the unknown
I learn to breathe
In this love umbilical

She told me my nipples were ugly, and that's why I couldn't breastfeed. In those first moments, staring at this stranger called my son, I was overcome with sadness and frustration. Women are sometimes the most hurtful critics of other women. I can't remember that nurse's name, but I do remember wishing that the anesthesia would wear off and allow me the freedom to connect my foot with whatever body part I could reach.

I phoned my doula crying and pleading for assistance. I'd been preparing for months to have a natural birth, and my body had not complied. I was disappointed.

Lying in a public hospital outside of my comfort zone was surreal, and the privacy of my thoughts was shattered by sharing a room with other mothers who themselves were far from the mirror of joy. This was supposed to be the happiest moment in my life. I had given another being a body and should have been proud, yet all I felt was fear.

Chapter 2: Myths and Barriers

My pregnancy was beautiful. I knew the process better than anyone. The dreams of my son's foretold coming, including the day of his conception, his gender, and his name. This was all gifted to me by my God and needed no intervention from any person or institution. It seemed as if all lines to the divine were now down. How was I going to nurture him if he didn't latch to the breast? I stared at the bottle at the side of my bed. It looked unclean and the milk suspect. Where was it from, who made it, and when? I wasn't breastfed as an infant. The connection I have with my own mother is non-existent in energy or memory.

My insecurities swallowed all the air in the room, yet I was still breathing. I was looking forward to breastfeeding. To making food for my child and passing down my immunity to him as I did not intend to vaccinate him. I also wanted to experience that oxytocin feel-good rush that my mother's friends kept raving about. I looked into my son's eyes—new, yet all-knowing—in search for some understanding. In their depth, I found the courage to keep trying.

When the anesthetic had worn off, I got up and left my sense of failure lying there alone to fend for itself. I found a teaspoon, tea cup, the kettle of boiling water, and headed back to my bed where I had left my son lying. I sterilized the spoon the best I could, and expressed colostrum from both breasts to spoon feed him.

The exercise was a success. Over the next few hours, we spoon fed and I continued to try breastfeeding without success as he struggled to latch. In between we cried together and slept as much as we could. I was afraid to let go of him, so he slept in my arms and woke up to my questioning eyes staring deeply into him.

He was born at 1:30 in the afternoon on a Monday. At about three in the morning on Tuesday after I had another cry, this time alone, I lay down to sleep with him held tightly to my breasts and he found his own way and latched.

That moment, I felt like I had just given birth. My son was eating and I felt completely fulfilled.

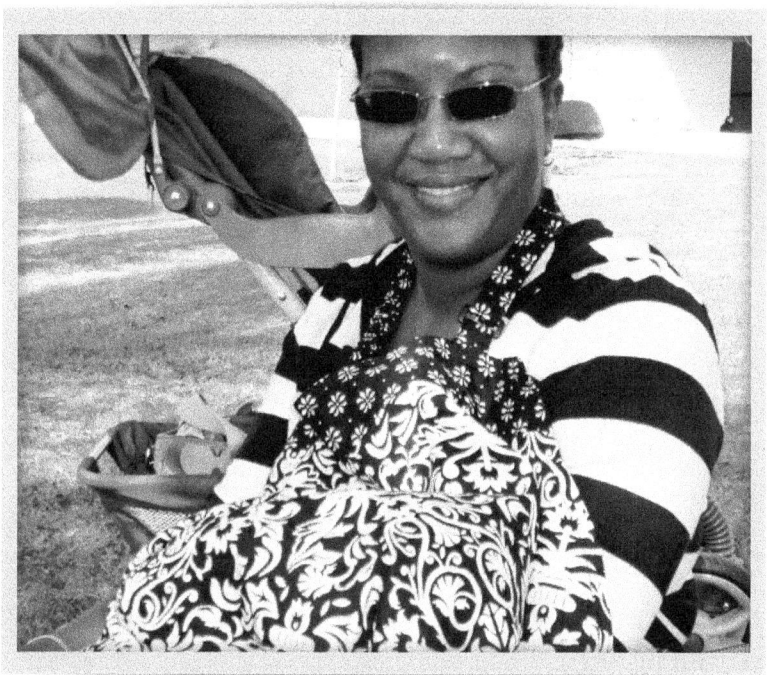

Breastfeeding in Public
by Natalie D. Preston-Washington

My oil change became due while on maternity leave. I tried to schedule it in between feedings, but like everything else, life rarely goes according to plans, especially when a baby is involved. Soon after arriving at the dealership, Luke started getting antsy. We walked around the new car lot—inside and out.

The change of scenery lasted about 10 minutes before I was soaked from sweat and he was looking for something more. He wanted milk and I had about five minutes to make it happen before it was on!

I approached the receptionist on the car floor and told her of my need. She suggested that I use a salesman's cubicle at the far end of the showroom.

Luke and I journeyed south and set up camp. As luck would have it, a salesman and customer approached. They were within earshot looking at a new vehicle. I am sure they saw me—the black and cream patterned nursing cover is hard to miss—but paid us no attention.

Whew! I moved Luke to the other side, careful not to flash the salesman and customer and whomever may be lurking behind me or on the other side of the glass wall.

Ring. My service advisor was calling. He needed to discuss an issue with my truck.

*Of course…*He sat across from me, maintaining eye contact. He has cared for my vehicle for years; knew me before I had a husband and baby, yet it was still a little odd to breastfeed in front of him. We talked, he called my husband on my behalf for his input, and all business was transacted without a peep show. Thankfully, Luke was really hungry and didn't have time to play and swat at the nursing cover! After that experience, I felt comfortable to nurse wherever and whenever the need presented itself.

Over the course of our 13-month breastfeeding era, I nursed in:
- *an airplane,*
- *a public park,*
- *a Baptist church,*

Chapter 2: Myths and Barriers

- *numerous restaurants,*
- *the back seat of my truck,*
- *the shopping mall sitting area,*
- *my office while meeting with my boss (a family medicine doctor and single mom of four), and*
- *all under the guise of my trusty nursing cover.*

It's coincidental that ABCs ethical dilemma series, *What You Do?*, ran a segment on breastfeeding in public—to a not-so receptive audience—during the same time that I was breastfeeding.

I watched it and was appalled at the treatment the nursing mother received. Thankfully, the nursing mother was an actress, but the ignorant naysayers were not. I guess God was looking out for me because I was never made to feel uncomfortable or unwelcome when I breastfed in public. Had someone approached me in the wrong manner, I would have educated them on the law that allows me to legally breastfeed in public, before I told them to back the fuck away from me and my baby.

No Fear
by Kahlillah Dotson Mosley

These are two separate posts that I wrote on an online mommy community. The change from one to the other in both my confidence as a nursing mom, and my grandparents' acceptance of my nursing, makes me proud.

They Hurt My Feelings – VENT 5.26.2009
So I went to visit the grandparents on this Memorial Day weekend. My whole family knows that I breastfeed. We go to Cracker Barrel and Khyri starts crying. He's two months old. He's hungry. So I discreetly pull out my cover and begin to breastfeed him....My grandfather leans over and says, *"Don't you want to do that in the car?"* My feelings were SO hurt. I politely got up and went to the car. I haven't felt any bad stares or stuff from anyone else—and I nurse in public all the time—so I was really hurt when my Grandpa said something.

When we were outside, I told Khyri to never be ashamed of anything. I may be sad, but I am not ashamed that I am choosing to feed my child the best milk possible. Hmph. So, to all of my fellow nursing mommies: Keep going!

Nursing In Public—No Fear 5.21.2011
We're here! We just completed our three-day road trip from Georgia to Virginia. I was able to make it sanely and in one piece—thank goodness! Yesterday we went to the Jubilee and had a GREAT time. It was so hot out there. Khyri had a great time!

Little Miss Kielle was a little overwhelmed. Maybe this was too much for a 3-month-old. I ran into a fellow nursing momma though, and that made me happy. I took both kiddos to the snack pavilion, and while Khyri was munching on grapes, I pulled the stroller in front of me and began to nurse Kielle.

I don't use a cover up anymore; this is baby #2. I'm comfortable in my own skin. There were a couple of stares, but then one mommy said to her toddler, *"Look she's nursing just like you used to."* It made me smile.

We got to talking and apparently her daughter had a hard time weaning, and just gave up the boob about two weeks earlier.

My grandma and grandpa came by and started chatting with us. I couldn't believe it. I thought they would walk right by and pretend they didn't see me. LOL. To my surprise, my grandma actually said she thinks it's good women are going back to nursing! That made me smile too.

Breastfeeding on My Time
by Tangela Walker-Craft

I decided to breastfeed my daughter until she was 2 years old. I was the first person in my family to practice what is called "extended breastfeeding" since the introduction of baby formula.

I thought this was a personal decision, between me and my husband and my child. But boy was I wrong.

I taught her a few baby signs by the time she was about 9 months old, so she knew how to tell me when she wanted to be nursed. During the first year she was exclusively breastfed. By the second year, she had a diet consisting of breast milk and toddler-appropriate foods. During her second year, she breastfed less than the year before.

Unfortunately, unwanted and unwelcomed advice on when I should wean her came from everywhere. People that have never breastfed a day in their lives will offer their advice about when's the best time to wean YOUR baby. Even people that have never had a child will somehow know when you've breastfed long enough. Unbelievable!

If you resist their unsolicited advice, people may even switch from asking when you plan to wean to trying to scare you into weaning. You'll likely hear, *"If you don't wean her soon, you won't be able to do it."* You may even get the, *"She's going to start biting you when she gets teeth,"* threat. It's funny how most people accept that a baby will start to walk when he or she is ready, and talk when he or

Chapter 2: Myths and Barriers

she is ready, but they think that there is a magic age when all babies should stop being breastfed. Once threats don't manage to scare you into submission, the attempts to shame you into weaning may begin. You'll get the loaded, *"You STILL breastfeeding that child? How old is she?"*

Family members and other people who feel they can will make snide remarks about how your child might be driving, married, or doing something else that's totally ridiculous before you wean him or her.

Things were particularly challenging because breastfeeding, especially extended breastfeeding, is not necessarily encouraged in Black families.

Like many breastfed babies, my daughter lacked the "baby bloat" that frequently occurs in formula-fed babies. My well-meaning grandmother asked me dozens of times if I was sure my baby was getting enough to eat. She'd ask me, *"Are you sure you're making enough milk?"*

She and other members of my family refused to believe that my baby could survive on just breast milk. I was constantly guarding against my family's threats to give my daughter "real food": formula.

After breastfeeding six children of her own out of necessity, my 85-year-old grandmother seemed to view my decision to voluntarily breastfeed as something outdated or odd. I think that moms that do not practice extended breastfeeding sometimes secretly resent moms that do.

There is a competitive spirit that makes women want other women to make the same childcare decisions that they've made. Women who do not, or did not, practice extended breastfeeding, may feel that moms who do are judging them for their choice.

Contrary to the warnings, weaning for me was easy. Taking natural cues from my daughter during that second year, I breastfed less and less during the daytime.

Breastfeeding became more of a bonding-and-comfort activity for us at night. When I sensed that she was ready, I began telling her that mommy wouldn't have any more milk soon. My breasts naturally responded by producing less milk because of the less-frequent feedings.

My daughter's nursing slowed down to a few minutes, only at bed time. Over a three-day period, I cut the feedings down to quick bouts, which culminated in the end of what was one of the best experiences of my life.

I am glad I never succumbed to the pressure to wean before we were ready, but it bothers me that such pressure exists. Why are we so uncomfortable with extended breastfeeding?

Chapter 3

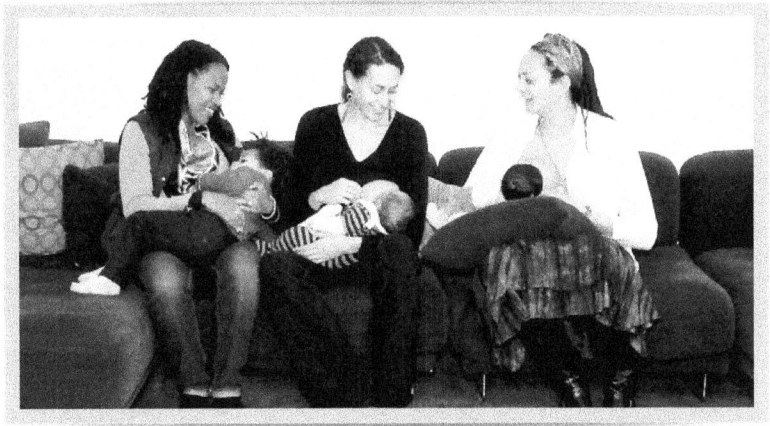

Healthy Mama, Thriving Baby

As these mothers nursed, they discovered the depths of this connection. Beyond the important statistics about reducing risks for breast cancer, SIDS, and obesity, there is a sacred connection between a healthy mother and a thriving baby. Support for breastfeeding means attention to the family: emotionally, physically, and spiritually.

Chapter 3: Healthy Mama, Thriving Baby

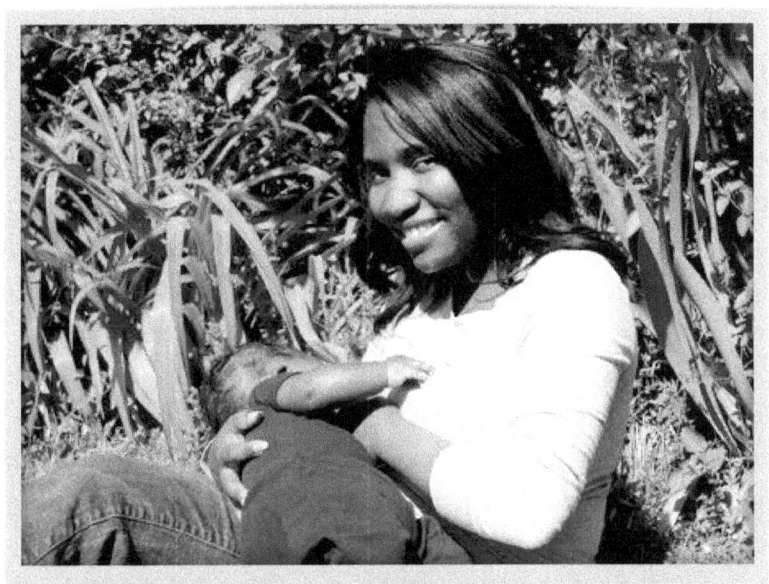

Celeste and Isaiah: Brown Mamas Breastfeed

I have been nursing for 11 weeks and plan to go until he self weans. I choose to breastfeed because that is what God made breasts for and it is the best for my son.

One thing I love about breastfeeding is when I look at how much he has grown, I know it is because of my milk. It makes me proud!

The Breastaurant Offers the Best Seat in the House
by Kinyofu Mlimwengu

Located near the heart of all mothers, is a quaint, yet attractive set of fine dining experiences for all babies. Easily accessible and conveniently located, The Breastaurant provides 24-hour meal preparation and effortless delivery. Whether the mother is at home or on the street, the internationally acclaimed Breastaurant is there to produce exactly what the child needs, in the exact quantity needed.

The Breastaurant is always prepared to offer the appropriate servings. Offering the contents of two breasts, eight to twelve times a day for the newborn; and later on ten to twelve times a day for the older baby, the Breastaurant is always super fresh and ready to serve. A mutual exchange is the norm, as the Breastaurant's main course keeps the baby hydrated; and the baby, as a regular consumer, keeps the Breastaurant well supplied. The Breastaurant makes sure the baby gets what it needs and even takes into account growth spurts, by creating more food as the child grows.

The frequency of feedings establishes a special closeness between mother and baby and becomes a true bonding experience. Furthermore, this sanctuary provides an intimate family experience as part of its ambiance. Daddy's joy is leaning on mommy's shoulder while marveling at the expression as his little one receives Nature's best. The Breastaurant brings forth an-age old, time-proven reinforcement of love, reassurance, and verbal pleasantries, with an overall feeling of satiation and self-assurance between the family triad, and also leads to a good night's sleep.

Chapter 3: Healthy Mama, Thriving Baby

More than a social tradition, the Breastaurant is sure to include just the right combination of protein and carbohydrates to support the baby's developing brain. The special, homemade preparation provides a unique cocktail of hormones, vitamins, and minerals—all originating from the best and most natural source of organic, chemical-free, and intuitively tailored ingredients to build on the baby's overall health.

One very distinctive element of the Breastaurant is its defense against disease due to the live antibacterial and antiviral cells included in the Breastaurant's cuisine. Also notable are the many discovered and undiscovered bonuses that not only improve the health of the baby, but also that of the mother.

Babies welcome the Breastaurant as a clear preference above all other alternatives as they do not offer the same special nuances. These highly publicized so-called alternatives are only weak imitations.

- *Legendary fine dining*
- *Internationally acclaimed*
- *Constantly changing*
- *Organic food production*
- *Breakfast, lunch, dinner, and snacks*
- *No recycling needed*
- *Made fresh daily*
- *Delivered fresh and natural*
- *Homemade*
- *Easily accessible*
- *A haven for the older child*

- *Serves only the best*
- *Carefully prepared to exalt the flavor of the family's cuisine*
- *A social tradition*
- *Invites intimate exchanges between mom/baby pair, and even dad*
- *Occasional oversized packaging*
- *Green*
- *Holistic*
- *Wholesome*
- *Customized*

Formula Feeding? Not for My Baby: One Mom's Story
by Tangela Walker-Craft

According to my Random House dictionary, definition No. 6 for the word *"formula"* is a mixture of milk and other ingredients for feeding a baby. I can deal with the milk; it's the other ingredients that concern me.

The word "formula" immediately makes me think of mad scientists hovering over test tubes in a laboratory. It also makes me think of experimenting and trial and error. Why "formulate" something to feed your baby when God has equipped most women's bodies to produce milk after they give birth? Breast milk has exactly the right amount of fat, sugar, water, and protein that a baby needs.

I once heard that humans are the only mammals that intentionally feed their young something other than their own milk. That, among many other factors, helped me decide not to give my baby formula. When breastfeeding is an option, I think Black mothers owe it to themselves and their babies to breastfeed for as long as possible. Other than women with illnesses that prevent them from breastfeeding, new moms should at least make an attempt to give their babies the considerable health advantages that breast milk has been proven to provide.

Extended breastfeeding has been credited with protecting babies from various illnesses. It is said to increase a child's intelligence, and it may also help prevent obesity. It is said that breastfeeding may offer protection from SIDS (Sudden Infant Death Syndrome). Some research has even linked the failure to breastfeed to intestinal issues experienced later in life. Breastfeeding exclusively for the first six months seems to offer babies significant health protection.

Moms benefit just as much from extended breastfeeding as their babies do. Breastfeeding moms are often free of a menstrual cycle for a longer period of time after giving birth. Breast, uterine, ovarian, and endometrial cancer risks are lower in women who practice extended breastfeeding. Diabetes is a disease that is prominent in the Black community. According to some studies, breastfeeding may lower insulin needs in diabetic women.

Weight loss is another incentive for extended breastfeeding. In my case, about three months into breastfeeding, I weighed less than I weighed prior to my pregnancy.

Along with the health benefits, extended breastfeeding provides an opportunity to bond with your baby in a way that no one else can. I can't put into words the joy I felt cradling my baby knowing that I was created by God to be able to nourish her. Mothers and babies are physically connected for 40 weeks during the baby's development. For breastfeeding mothers and babies, extended nursing is a continued physical, emotional, and spiritual link.

A Life Changing Event: Accounts from My Diary
by Monica Z. Utsey

A Premature Birth
I went into preterm labor on Monday, April 24th. I arrived at the hospital around 11:30 p.m. fully expecting to have the labor stopped and go home on bed rest. I was scared, but never thought in a million years that I would deliver my child. I didn't know it, but I had been in labor since about 7 p.m. By 5:30 a.m. on Tuesday, April 25th, the doctors told me *"this baby is coming."*

I delivered him at 9:54 a.m. that morning, at 28 weeks. He was not due until July 20. At this point I kind of blanked out and went into denial because *"this couldn't really be happening."*

The whole experience was the complete opposite of almost everything I believe in. I was given morphine, magnesium sulfate, insulin, antibiotics, and more drugs. I labored flat on my back, hooked up to all kinds of machines, and a perfect stranger delivered my baby. Now compare this to the kind of birth I intended—a calming, water birth with a midwife that I had developed a relationship with over a period of 10 months. Big difference!

Over the last few weeks, I've had to reframe my perception of this event into a more positive and thankful one. I've also gained a profound respect for modern medicine. And, by the grace of God's mercy, my son is here and he's alive. The neonatologist on duty that night happened to be a very tender doctor of Indian descent, Dr. Cherian at Washington Hospital Center, who calmed all of my fears and assured me that my son would be fine. Through the entire ordeal, my husband Eric, never left my side and advocated for me in every way. Claudia Booker (she would have been my birthing assistant at the Birth Center) came and made me feel like a queen, and showed those nurses how I was supposed to be treated after giving birth.

I was terrified after giving birth, but when they told me he weighed 3 lbs. 2oz. I was a bit more optimistic. I went into labor totally ignorant about preemies. The doctor assured me that preemies in his condition had a survival rate of 90%. I just cried. My son's Godmother arrived in time to pray right before I gave birth. She took Zion, my 6-year-old son, downstairs to the cafeteria for breakfast, and by the time they returned, his little brother was here. Then Corliss called and prayed with me (thank you!).

Then Momma Teresa showed up, followed by my Pastor and his wife. So instead of crying my eyes out, I was surrounded by people who prayed over me. But it was still hard. My Pastor prayed over me and said today is a joyous occasion because some mothers carry a baby for 10 months and deliver a stillborn. He said your son is here and he is alive. This became my new paradigm for his birth.

After seeing my baby for the first time, I was afraid to be alone. I didn't know how I would make it. How could I go home and function? My first thought was will he live and the next was will I be able to breastfeed. And each time I had resigned myself to come back to my room and cry my eyes out, there was a beautiful Mocha Mom sitting in the visitor's chair with food, encouraging words, and a smile. I will never ever forget your presence for as long as I live. It is because of you that I was able to make it through the two days at

Chapter 3: Healthy Mama, Thriving Baby

the hospital. Leaving the hospital empty-handed was probably the worst. I spent the first two weeks crying.

Then after a conversation with another sister friend, Althea, who is a medical intuitive, I realized that I had to steel myself for the road ahead. Because of my sisters, I was able to focus on loving my son, eating, sleeping, praying, and pumping. Now, my milk supply is overflowing. I'm pumping more than 30 ounces of milk per day! Knowing that I will be able to breastfeed my son is keeping my spirits high.

It's still hard, and I have moments when I just cry. When I see a pregnant mom or a new baby, I slip into the *"why me?"* It's getting more and more difficult to go to the hospital every day, see my son, and then go home. But my faith is keeping me strong sometimes. They all say the life of a preemie in the NICU is up and down. So I never know what to expect. But I affirm only the positive.

When the time came for us to name him, I had to really accept him as mine. He was no longer this baby in the NICU, but my son: Ayinde Kamau Utsey. Ayinde is a Yoruba name from Nigeria, which means *"the son we prayed for"* or *"we gave praises and he came."* Kamau is a Kikuyu name from Kenya, which means *"quiet warrior."* Our family translates this to mean: *"The son we prayed for is a quiet warrior."*

The NICU (from my diary)
Yesterday, following Ayinde's birth, I was feeling discouraged because the nurses in the NICU told me that I brought in *"too much milk."* I'm pumping about 24 to 32 oz. bottles a day (three to

69

six bottles at each session and I pump about eight times per day). They showed me my storage supply, and it fills up two shelves in their freezer. They told me they have "never" seen a mother of a premature baby pump so much milk, and that I have enough milk there to feed the entire nursery for three months. They started suggesting that I donate some of my milk to a milk bank.

So they said that I could not bring in any more breast milk, and I had to take home some of the milk I had stored there. My freezer is full, my mother's freezer is full, and we don't have a deep freezer. So where is this milk going to go? They also told me that they could only supply me with 8-10 bottles a day, so now we have to go out and buy some of the plastic milk storage bags (which aren't as good as the bottles).

I guess I'm sensitive now, so I just came home and cried. I felt rejected and criticized. Then to make matters worse, they tried to imply that my milk was making the baby gassy.

When I do my 5 a.m. pumping, my milk supply is highest, so I'm able to pump enough milk to feed the baby for two days (six bottles. They can only use three, so I have to freeze three).

My husband takes this milk into the hospital by 6 a.m. each morning so the baby is now getting fresh milk each day instead of frozen milk that has been thawed. So now I have to be the "gas" police. Nevertheless, I'm willing to do whatever it takes so that Ayinde can have fresh milk because it's better for him, and I know that my body is constantly updating my milk with the antibodies he needs.

So as I go to visit him in the NICU, my body is producing antibodies to the germs in the NICU, and I can pass this protection on to my son via the breast milk. A woman's body is so awesome!

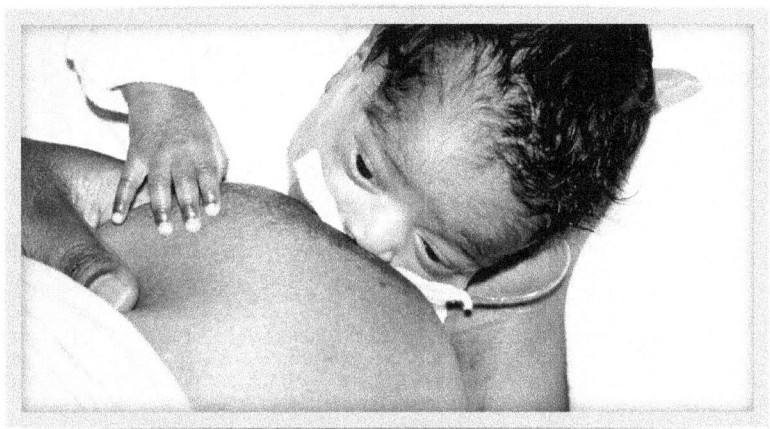

Breastfeeding—A Huge Success
Breastfeeding was my number one priority. I knew this would make a huge difference in my son's life with all of the possible issues that could lie ahead. I received a pamphlet while in the hospital on breastfeeding a preemie, and I followed it to a "tee." I pumped around the clock every two hours to mimic the feeding patterns of a newborn. I went to bed at midnight, and then I would wake at 5:00 a.m. and do the same thing.

I just returned home from spending my first entire night with my son in eight weeks! The HSC Pediatric Center has a parent apartment reserved for families to "practice" being at home with their child.

The reality of being the mother of a newborn hit me like a ton of bricks. The purpose of this overnight visit was to practice breastfeeding and caring for my son. I had to hook up his monitors, change diapers, hook up his tube feedings, the whole nine yards. Big UPs to the nurses! I have been up ALL NIGHT, literally.

But awakening to his sweet cry was such a blessing. Because Ayinde is not able to go to breast for each feeding (premature babies tire easily at the breast), I had to determine which feedings would be skipped, and which feedings require me to supplement him with my breast milk and tube syringe. And on top of all of that juggling, I still had to fit in pumping sessions to keep my supply up. Like Zion, Ayinde has a *"Kung Fu Grip Latch,"* but his mouth is too small to take in all of my areola, so sometimes he had fun gnawing on my nipple—ouch! But again, gazing down into those eyes made all the pain go away.

At one point during the evening, I sat on the edge of the bed and cried. Ayinde is not strong enough to empty my breasts so sometimes after a nursing session; he will need to be "topped off" with breast milk from a supplemental feeder. Eric and Zion were sleeping peacefully, and I was trying to figure out how to use the Medela SNS (Supplemental Nursing System), which I believe is impossible to do alone.

How in the heck do you tape the tube on your nipples without the milk dripping all over the place? When I tried to put Ayinde to breast, the tube kept sticking up his nose. So I just cried, put him back in the crib and hooked up his feeding syringe. I was tired and frustrated, and so was he.

Now I see how some moms say, *"Shoot, I'm a formula baby and I'm okay."* Heck, I'm a formula momma [formula fed as a baby]. But I know too much about breastfeeding's benefits to turn back now. I am affirming that he will be getting all of his nourishment from my breast. Please affirm that with me.

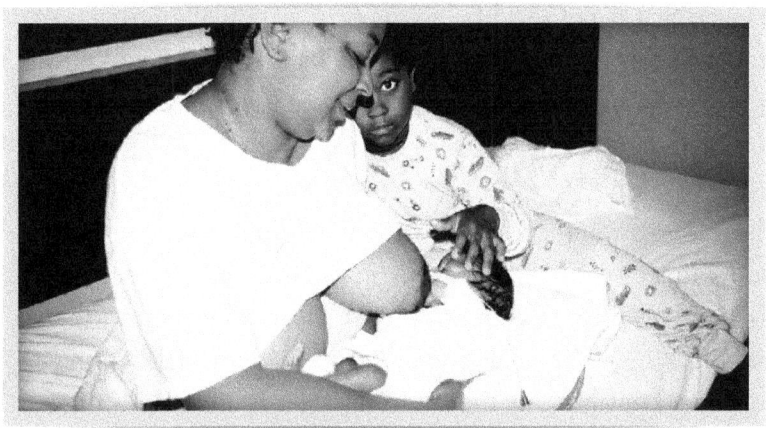

My 5-Year-Old
If I had to pick one word to describe Ayinde it would be "determined." It is such a joy to share his world. He is such a creative and intelligent young child. He loves music and dance. He has been studying violin since he was 3-years-old and African drums since he was 4-years-old. I am so blessed to help guide him in the journey of life.

Feeding a Nation
by Tiffany Gorman

The day I found out I was pregnant was one of the happiest moments in my life. I immediately began planning her birth. I am a planner, I like things to go according to my plan, but as we all know that is not real life. So my plan was an all-natural water birth, where my baby is handed to me bloody and all and nurses for the first time. Aww, I wanted the total hippie, crunchy granola, motherland experience.

I received an induced labor with an epidural, a little pushing, ending in a c-section. After being in the hospital for two days, no food, and now baby cut out of me, all I wanted was to nurse my newborn. One hour later I finally got to hold my little Amina Sunshine. I put her tiny mouth to my breasts and ouch! It felt a little weird and uncomfortable. A lactation specialist came in and helped me to get her to latch right, and we were good to go.

My next plan was to nurse for at least a year, longer if we both wanted to do it. The first week my left nipple had scabs all over it. So I let her nurse on the right side, which toughened up quickly, and pumped from the left until it was healed. That first time feeling my milk let down I truly understood why I had breasts. Not to be big in dresses, or fun bags for our partners, but to nourish a nation. It was the most significant action I had ever made toward humanity. I was feeding my child.

The ease of it was what I really loved. Anywhere we were, if she was hungry, I could feed her—for free—the best stuff on Earth. I fed her at the mall, the park, and restaurants. I noticed I received a lot of smiles from other moms, and stares from most others. Who cared about them?

As she got older, she would just nosedive toward a breast when she was in my arms. She fell asleep at night with me singing to her and nursing. She really started eating solids around 5 months, but was still nursing most of the time. She did take a bottle, because I pumped so my husband and others could feed her. But as a stay-at-home mother, I was able to feed her most of the time.

I went back to work when she was 10 months. With the stress of a new job, being away from her, and being a working mom, I just didn't produce as much milk as before. She was eating most meals and took a bottle of formula if I didn't have enough. But that was short lived, by age 1 she was drinking soymilk from a sippy cup and eating food.

I didn't get the 1+ year I was looking for, but I enjoyed the 10 months I had. Whenever I talk to a pregnant woman, I always ask if they plan on breastfeeding. I encourage young girls to breastfeed when they become mothers. It is beneficial in many ways. Yes, you are feeding your baby, but you are doing more: you are bonding in the most simple and profound way. Plus, you are treating your body right. Your milk is made from what you eat, so you will be more inclined to eat what is right. I understand the need and convenience of formulas but hospitals shouldn't hand it out as routine. Everyone should at least try nursing. Maybe you don't make enough milk, fine use the formula. But to never try is not using your breasts for what they were meant for—making milk.

Chapter 4

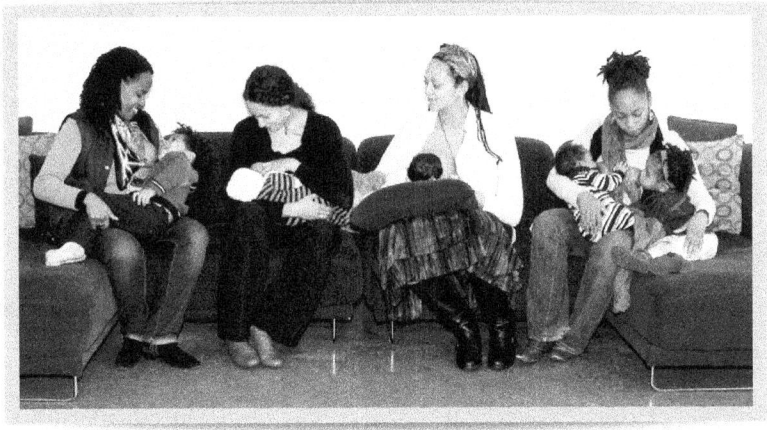

When the Bough Breaks

Discomfort, pain, and fear can happen. These are the reflections of mothers from their moment at the crossroads of uncertainty. Their stories make it clear that a support circle can be the deciding factor for whether or not a mother nurses.

Chapter 4: When the Bough Breaks

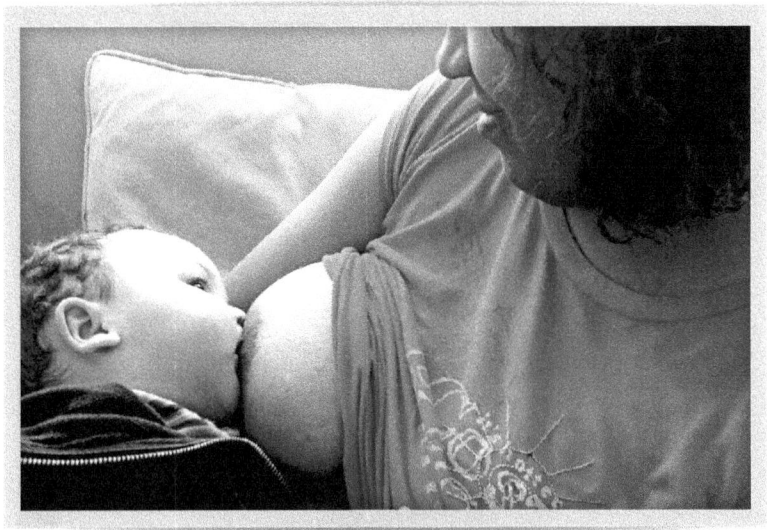

Sakinah and Maximo: Brown Mamas Breastfeed

Maximo was breastfed for 22 months. After the experience of breastfeeding his older brother for 18 months, nursing Maximo was very easy for me. There was an initial learning curve with the first child, but I stuck it out with support from my lactation consultant, Leigh Anne O'Connor, and with a lot of support from my husband.

I loved the closeness and the cuddling that happens when breastfeeding. Nursing became so easy once I had the hang of it. I thought of it as almost being lazy...at least I didn't have to fuss with bottles! I always had a way to soothe my baby no matter where we were, which was extremely convenient. I never worried about nursing in public, and did so whenever necessary and wherever my baby and I were comfortable.

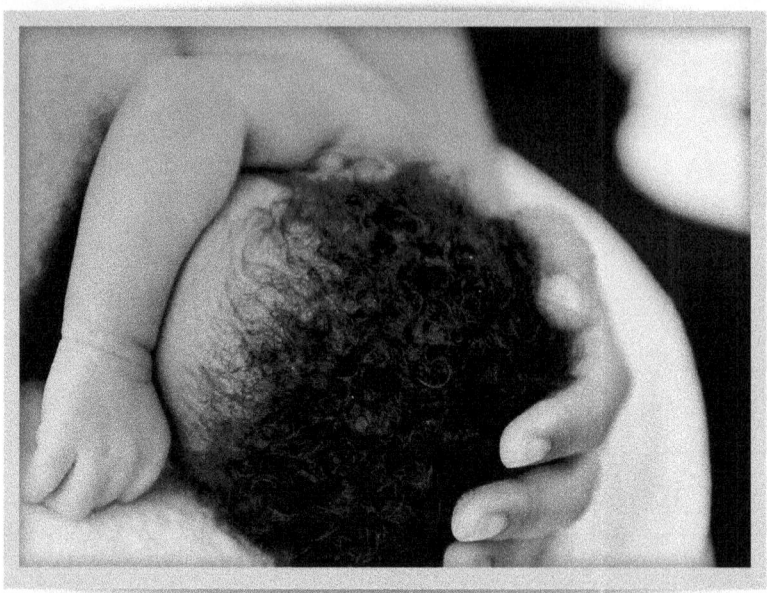

My Story
by Evvett Pickens

I am a first-generation breastfeeder to my baby, Isabella. I never knew about breastfeeding, and would have probably formula fed because that's all that I've ever seen.

One year, I had a friend give birth. She told me *"I breastfeed because it's free."* That's all she said, but it was the perfect thing for this cheapskate to hear!

When I became pregnant, two of my other friends breastfed, so I immediately thought, *"this must be easy."* I mean, the women in Africa on TV do it all of the time, right?! If you have a baby, and two boobs, it should be the easiest thing ever!

I really should have done my research.

When Isabella was born, my milk didn't come in. She initially weighed 7.7, but dropped down to 7.1 lbs. By the time, she went to her first doctor's appointment, she was 6.83! I cried and cried for about two days. I tried to get her to nurse, but she would fuss and punch my breasts.

One time, my mother (who was staying the night) burst into my room and accused me of trying to be like my friends, saying *"why don't you give that baby regular milk!"* I was so crushed. A couple of days later, I reached out to a lactation consultant. She immediately fixed Isabella's latch, and got me off of anything that could be making her fussy and colicky.

I found myself in a weekly support group where I was the only African American. I had to get over the uncomfortable feeling, because these women were giving me the support I needed. I couldn't, and still cannot locate an African-American support group in my area.

Now, Isabella is 6 months old and thriving! She loves to nurse and it's such a special moment for us! I tell the world that my African-American baby has been breastfed! I want everyone to know that they can come to me for questions or concerns, and that Black women do breastfeed!

Coming Full Circle
by Kiara Diggs

I had always known that I wanted to breastfeed my children, even when they were only a sweet dream in my young eyes. I saw what my mother went through with not having the opportunity to breastfeed me. She mentioned it often as I grew up, and I knew it saddened her. I wanted to be able to develop a wonderful connection with my baby and to be able to feed the baby naturally. Along with being a mother, that was always my wish.

So when I became pregnant with my firstborn in 2008, I carried those wishes with me. I didn't even blink at the thought; it was a given that I would breastfeed her. I prepared for her arrival in every other way. I had my midwife, planned the homebirth, looked for a home to purchase, and prepared myself to bring her into the world. The one thing that I didn't prepare for was breastfeeding.

I was naïve. I romanticized about how it would be. I thought that the baby just came out, latched onto my breast, and we would sail down the river of breastfeeding bliss. I went to my prenatal visits with an OB/GYN and my midwife, but didn't think to take any breastfeeding classes. I read several books, but none that were specific to the science and technique of breastfeeding.

My beautiful daughter was born in February 2009, and my fantasy of how breastfeeding would be for us quickly crumbled. I immediately noticed that it was uncomfortable, but I didn't really know how it was supposed to feel. My midwife assured me that some babies don't just come out ready to nurse, but that she had enough "reserves" to last her a little while. When I began to try to feed her consistently, it was as if she couldn't grasp my nipple.

A couple days after her birth, my midwife came back for a visit, and I shared with her that my baby didn't seem to latch on or get any milk out. She advised me that I wasn't putting my nipple in far enough; that the entire areola should be in her mouth. I tried to do as she suggested, but still didn't have much luck. It also became increasingly painful. After a couple days of the struggling, my baby became very weak and lethargic. As a new mother, I was deeply panicked. I kept thinking to myself, *"They don't tell you about all this stuff in the pregnancy books!"*

After a mastitis scare and my daughter's lethargy, my midwife suggested a lactation consultant. I didn't even know such a person existed. After assessing my daughter, she advised me to place my breastfeeding on hold and put my daughter on a rigorous diet to get her eating well. She had lost a considerable amount of weight and needed to gain it back. We used a finger feeding technique to make sure she was getting about 4 oz. of breast milk every two hours.

After my daughter recovered, I went back to trying to breastfeed her. It was so painful that it took me a few minutes before every feeding to even place my nipple in her mouth. I had to coax myself into doing it. The lactation consultant concluded that the difficulty was because my daughter's frenulum was too short and it limited her tongue's mobility. When a baby breastfeeds, the tongue sits under the nipple and it's what transports the milk into the mouth. It made sense to me because it felt like she was just "gumming" my nipple, but the only option to fix it was minor surgery.

My daughter's pediatrician assured me that she was not *"tongue-tied,"* and that she was latching on fine. With the uncertainty of it all, I just kept trying. And many times I would just give up. I continued the finger feeding too, and eventually went on to straight bottle feeding her with my milk. Between the constant pumping and complications with breastfeeding her directly, my nipples were cracked, burning, and scabbed; none of which seemed normal to me.

I also consulted many of my mommy friends. They too said that the pain was all a part of the process, and that my nipples had to adjust. There just wasn't much concern; it was if it was a rite of passage that every Mom had to go through. They kept reassuring me that the pain and discomfort wouldn't last. I began to question my own tolerance for pain, even though I labored with my daughter for 27 hours.

Once the pain turned into continual burning, I did my own research. I found out that burning, cracked, bloody nipples, and infections were all signs that the baby wasn't latching or positioned properly. I felt relieved because I knew I wasn't crazy and grew more confident in my lactation consultant's original assessment. I also found out that the burning was most commonly associated with thrush. I treated my nipples with gentian violet, and still tried to carry on. The pain didn't stop.

It wasn't until my mother came up for a visit, and heard me scream at the top of my lungs while holding onto her leg, that I snapped out of my unwavering attempts to breastfeed my baby. She told me that she knew how much I wanted to breastfeed my daughter, but that my experience wasn't normal. Not only was her well-being compromised because I was in such a frenzied state, but I needed to take care of myself emotionally. It was then that I realized that I needed to do something different. I had been torturing myself in order to maintain this ideal of breastfeeding my baby by any means necessary. And neither me nor my baby was at peace. I had to make one of the most difficult decisions of my life.

With the difficulty of breastfeeding, postpartum depression, and other various issues, I decided to put my baby on organic soy formula. She was only a couple months old. Many cringed at the thought, but at the time it was the best I could do. I was disappointed by what happened but, I still created opportunities for us to continue building our connection as mother and daughter.

When my baby was about 6 months old, I found out I was pregnant with my second baby. As hard at it was to accept that my dream of breastfeeding my daughter was deferred, I do believe that things turned out that way for a reason. It was almost as if my daughter knew he was coming before I did and was making room for his arrival. And from the moment I brought him home, I always said it was as if they knew each other before they got here.

My shining "sun" was born in May 2010, and to my heart's content, he latched on with ease. I read a breastfeeding guide beforehand, to ensure that I was well-equipped to handle any potential challenges. Of course, there was pain and I did develop thrush again on my right nipple, but it was pain that I could handle, and I was able to nurse my nipple back to health since I was already aware of the signs of thrush.

Breastfeeding my son, and experiencing the normalcy and the manageable pain, gave me more peace with the difficulty I had with my daughter. It was confirmation for me that there were definite issues with the level of pain I experienced.

I felt sad at times for not being able to have that same type of experience that I was having with my son, but the most important thing was that she was as beautiful and as healthy as ever. And she became a part of my breastfeeding experience with my son because she was always right there with us. And ironically, my son has had more minor health concerns than she has. Thankfully, my son had the pleasure of being breastfed exclusively (no bottles or pumps) until he was 7 months old, when he started some solids. Even after introducing him to foods, he still breastfed without bottles until he was 16 months old.

More peace and resolve came when my daughter was 2 years old. I took her to the dentist for her first visit, and unexpectedly found out that she did, in fact, have a short frenulum. She confirmed my lactation consultant's assessment, and I could rest easier knowing that it wasn't something that I was doing wrong.

I share my story because it sheds light on the importance of breastfeeding awareness, education, and support. I am a mother who advocates for breastfeeding, and practices natural living in all aspects of our lives. By no means am I saying that formula is the way; I fully believe in mother's milk.

But my journey brought me to a place where at the time, I had to use it. I know a lot more about other viable options now than I did back then. What my situation helped me to see is that given my lifestyle, if I was unaware, there may be countless other mothers out there in similar situations. They may want to breastfeed, and have every intention to, but without proper guidance and support, will give up if issues arise.

When you feel alone, uncertain, and overwhelmed, it can become easier to resort to formula feeding. There is also a great divide between mothers who breastfeed and mothers who choose to formula feed. Just as we breastfeeding mothers would like for people to recognize the beauty of what is a natural process; we have to educate people with love and positivity, instead of criticism and negativity. We also need to take more time to understand people's reasoning so that we can better address the underlying issues there.

It is my hope that through this movement, more Black women will have access to breastfeeding education, preparation classes, and continual breastfeeding support. Many women who breastfeed live a certain lifestyle, and the resources linger amongst very specific mommy groups.

If we are to reach the masses—particularly in underserved and poverty-stricken communities—we need to not only empower women to embrace breastfeeding, but to also see to it that they have the resources to make it through the potential difficulties. I am wishing all the mothers out there, beautiful, easy, and successful breastfeeding journeys!

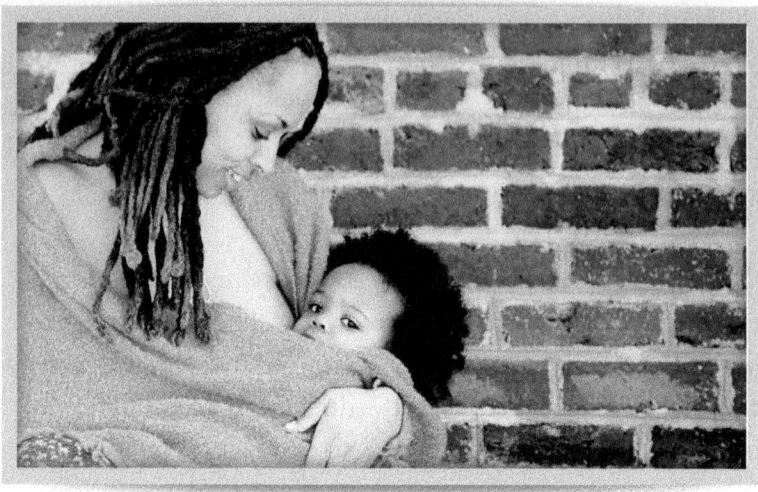

Learning Sacrifice
by Tracy Eleazer

It is such an empowering experience to know that your body was designed in a way to nurture and sustain life through breastfeeding. I couldn't imagine not using my God-given ability to provide the added benefits of breastfeeding for my child and me.

Breastfeeding for me did not *"magically"* happen. It did not come without its challenges. Breastfeeding requires commitment, dedication, sacrifice and energy. I was intimately familiar with sore, cracked nipples, and engorgement. Among other things, I have nursed through sickness, nausea, sore nipples, exhaustion and although it wasn't easy, I did it and survived. How does the old adage go? *"What doesn't kill you makes you stronger."*

The process was constant, and sometimes wearing, especially when I added pumping to the equation, however, it is just one of the many sacrifices that we as mothers make. Knowing that I am providing my child with the best nourishment possible is reason enough for me.

Breastfeeding for me was not just physical. It was a spiritual and emotional journey. The amazing bond between mother and child that is created seems *"magical."* I think breastfeeding is an extension of our body's ability to give birth.

Breastfeeding for me has been love: priceless, precious, empowering, challenging, comforting, emotional, fulfilling, and a blessing all wrapped up into one!

The longest that I've breastfed any one of my children has been two years, with another *"blessing"* on the way. I will just allow it to happen. I applaud all mothers who breastfeed and give of themselves unconditionally.

I can't thank my husband enough for his continued support. Like I said, breastfeeding did not come without its challenges, but he was always right there by my side encouraging me, lifting me up, and saying what a wonderful job I was doing.

He never once questioned my body's ability to produce the *"liquid gold."* He never suggested that I give up and offer the baby formula. Together we found a way to continue, *"To fight the good fight,"* and for that I am grateful!

Breastfeeding, for me, has been a journey, but definitely one worth taking!

Four Days
by Ambata Kazi-Nance

Day One.   *Monday, June 22, 2009*
4:24 a.m. My son's first cry brings tears of relief to my eyes. He's here. My son is born. And I, his mother, am born too. A brief glimpse of my son and then he is whisked away. My husband goes with him and I am left alone on the operating table. My body is numb, and I have never felt so tired. Nurses and doctors talk to me, but I am too tired to speak, the effort of opening my mouth is too exhausting. I sink into the bright lights above my head and drift off to sleep.

5:30 a.m. Sun peeking through the blinds. The door opens and finally my son is brought to me. The nurse places him in my waiting arms. The feelings are indescribable. Here is the child that has lived in me for the past nine months. My husband, the nurse, and my midwife surround me, expectantly. I feel they are waiting for me to do something, but I'm not sure what. I am so confused, so tired, my mind foggy from the epidural given before the surgery. Finally the nurse asks me if I would like to feed my son. Feed him? Me? Yes, I want to, but I have no idea how.

I sit there with my son in my arms, dumbfounded. All that I read and all that I know have escaped my brain. My husband helps me loosen my gown, and I bring my son to my breast, feeling awkward, sure that I am doing it all wrong. I look to the nurse and the midwife for help. They look back with kind, encouraging smiles. I look down to my son, hoping he will know what to do, but he seems as clueless as me. He takes a few tentative sucks and then moves away. I feel a panic coming on, but the nurse and midwife assure me that when he is hungry he will nurse.

I am relieved to be done with this moment, this feeling of inadequacy, wanting to hide my face from embarrassment. Drunk from pain medications, I spend much of the day like this, drifting in and out of consciousness, barely able to greet the family and friends who come to visit. Idris and I are off to a bumpy start with breastfeeding, but for now we are riding the waves.

Day Two.   *Tuesday, June 23, 2009*
9 p.m. Another day of visitors and fumbling attempts at breast-feeding. Those waves are getting rockier and rockier. My calm, sleepy baby boy is getting hungry. Colostrum isn't satisfying him. My husband has gone home to shower and gather a few changes of clothes. Idris is hungry, and I don't know what to do.

"My baby will only have my breast milk." This has been my pledge for the past nine months. But my milk isn't here yet. His cries pierce my heart. The nurses are coming every hour. Has he had any wet diapers? Has he had a bowel movement? No. They are kind, but their questions increase the panic that is growing inside me. What do I do? He won't stop crying. I give him my breast, and he sucks a few times, then cries louder. I call a nurse. I am fighting back tears. I don't know what to do. I don't know how to soothe my child. The nurse asks, gently, if I want to try some formula. No! My baby will only have my breast milk. Idris's cries increase. We reach a compromise. With a small cup, I pour a few drops of formula into Idris's mouth.

His cries stop. He is silent. He smacks his lips with satisfaction. I bring him back to my breast and feed him formula through a syringe while he nurses. Relief floods over me. The tension in the air vanishes. I am disappointed, but still determined. A little formula will not interfere with my plans. My son will still have my breast milk.

Day Three.   *Wednesday, June 24, 2009*
The lactation nurse is here to help. She shows me how to use an electric breast pump to stimulate milk production. She teaches me different positions that make nursing easier. I am introduced to the football hold, a hold I will use for many months in the future.

My milk hasn't arrived yet, but I am feeling more confident after talking to the lactation nurse. She assures me I am doing everything right, and makes me feel proud that I am choosing to breastfeed my baby. Bringing my son to my breast is beginning to feel more natural and a lot less clumsy.

Day Four.   *Thursday, June 25, 2009*
Liquid Gold! My milk has arrived, and the floodgates cannot hold it back. Along with my milk comes a tremendous wave of emotions. I spend most of the day crying; crying because we are parents now, crying because I am a mother, crying because my body aches in ways I never knew possible, crying because I don't know why I keep crying. Idris cries too, but now bringing him to my breast stops his tears instead of increasing them. *"We are now attached in a way that seems closer even than when he was in utero."*

Though the milk flowed generously from then on, there were still many bumps over those two years I breastfed my son. The first three weeks were painful, as I dealt with sore, tender nipples, back pains from milk production, and general postpartum aches and pains. There were times during those first few weeks when I had to close my eyes and say a prayer before bringing my son to my breast because it hurt so badly. I can say though that I was not tempted to give up on breastfeeding.

My husband and I had intended two things even before I got pregnant that we would have a natural, non-medicated birth, and that I would breastfeed our child. My son's birth was out of my hands, of course. Complications due to fibroids blocking the birth canal led to an emergency c-section. But my feelings on both our intentions were strong; I didn't give up my plans for a natural birth without a fight. And I fought just as hard to breastfeed and was successful.

Breastfeeding wasn't always easy, but I wouldn't have it any other way. Through my son, and through breastfeeding, I have learned what selflessness and unconditional love are really all about. All the pain, all the tears, the long hours, the late-night feedings; all of it was worth it.

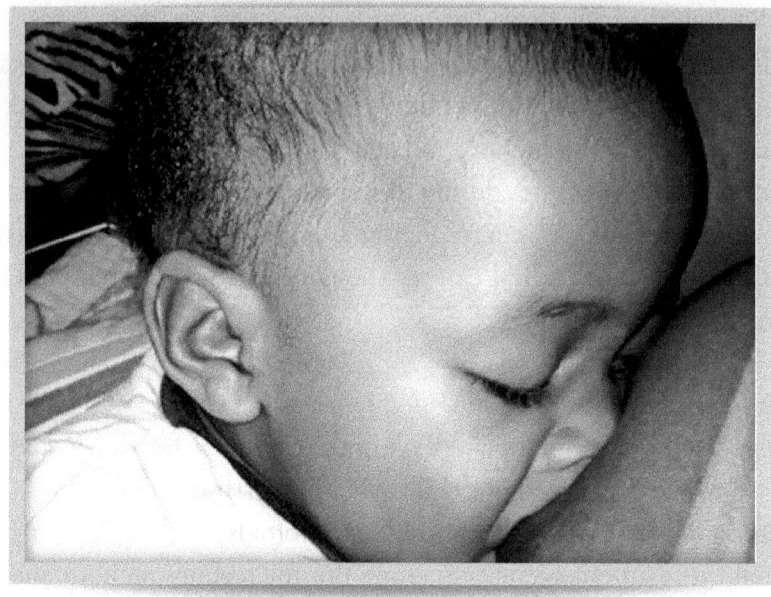

Breastfeeding Support
by Natalie D. Preston-Washington

It was never a question of *"if,"* but one of *"how long"* I would breastfeed. Since conception, I knew that would be the route for my baby.

I worked in a college of public health, and was surrounded by educators who promoted the benefits of a mother's milk. In fact, I was naïve enough that I did not even entertain the difficulties that would arise, and I committed to three months without hesitation. The only reason I did not commit to longer initially was because my breasts were my "go-to" erogenous zone. I wanted to wait and see how long (and how well) I could tolerate "my girls" being off-line.

Well, once Luke arrived on the scene, extreme fatigue, round-the-clock parenting, and zero desire was enough to sideline "my girls" for awhile. So, if I could make it work, Luke was entitled to all that I could produce. I recall standing in the hospital bathroom, reveling at my newfound stripper tits. My milk was in, and I was excited. At least until I tried to sleep that night. It was torture.

My breasts and back were in extreme pain, and I had to secure a pain reliever to rest semi-comfortably. At home, I was confused. Everything I read said don't over pump or you will produce more milk. Clearly, "my girls" were producing too much milk, but how would I get rid of it? Luke and I were still trying to get the hang of nursing. Even our best try resulted in short bouts of feeding, and this was literally too much for him to swallow anyway.

It was Sunday morning, and my outpatient lactation consultant was not available. I consulted with a coworker and good friend who suggested I try La Leche League. There were five or six ladies listed for my region. After getting several voicemails, I was down to the last person. She answered. *"Hallelujah!"*

We talked for what seemed like hours. She e-mailed me literature and links to how-to videos online. Thanks to La Leche League, I survived my initial engorgement and subsequent bouts with thrush.

Over the next few months, I became intimately familiar with clogged milk ducts. It seems that my plethora of milk liked to hang out on the inside, too. I remember one round of clogs that was particularly bad. I sent my hubby to SuperTarget to secure cabbage leaves. I massaged the problem areas until my hand was sore.

I wasted gallons of streaming water in the shower. Nothing worked.

I reached out to the same coworker and friend who referred me to La Leche League, and she shared what she did with her children.

The baby would be on the floor. She hovered over and let *"her girls"* dangle over the baby's mouth. The baby was then able to nurse, and *"the girls"* were free of any obstruction and pressure. Picture a mother animal feeding her young in the wild. Okay, I admit it sounds weird. But it works. At least it worked for me! From that point on, any clogged duct was treated with the same regimen.

A girlfriend was visiting from Virginia when Luke was about 1 ½ months old. She had just arrived at our home. My husband let her in. She climbed the stairs, and there I was on the living room floor, topless and hovering over a hungry baby. No shame in my game. The clog needed to be gone, and that was priority number one!

Of course, I dealt with nipples that were sore to the touch and a few other things, but they pale in comparison to engorgement, thrush, and clogged ducts.

Without a support system, I doubt Luke and I would have lasted the initial three months.

So, to my:
- *Local La Leche League volunteers*
- *Mommy coworkers group*
- *Friends with young kids*

- *Outpatient lactation consultant*
- *Students who are lactation consultants*
- *God*
- *And, countless others*

Thank you for the support, knowledge imparted, resources shared, and overall kindness and understanding that allowed me to breastfeed my son for 13 wonderful (in hindsight) months!

Chapter 5

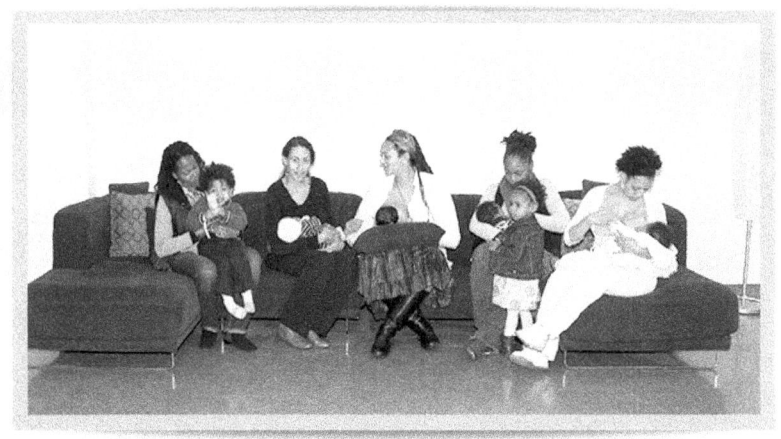

Breastfeeding Warriors

*There are challenges...
and there are battles.
In the following
reflections,
you will hear
from women
about overcoming
major life circumstances
to continue
breastfeeding, and
women who
provided their milk
for multiple babies,
even ones they
did not birth.*

Chapter 5: Breastfeeding Warriors

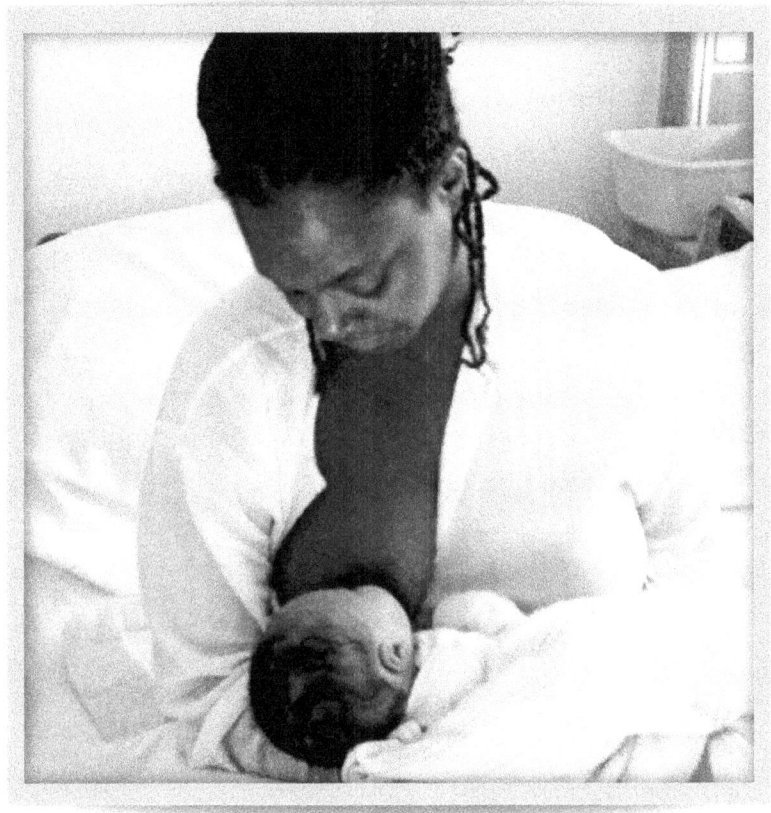

Since the beginning of time
by Tina Mooney

I breastfed two of my children until their 5th birthdays. Extended nursing and tandem nursing were never anything that I needed to think twice about doing. For me, it just seemed like a natural progression: you get pregnant, then the baby comes out of you and goes right into your arms. And then, there are breasts that are full of food. End of story. It really was that simple for me.

If I was holding a baby in arms then the natural thing to do was put him on the breast. When I was younger and having my first children, I didn't know about nutrition, health benefits, or even the psychological benefit of bonding that came from breastfeeding. All I knew was that it was a relationship I wanted to enjoy. I also had no idea that I would do it for five full years. I could probably have gone on forever, but the feedings were becoming farther and farther between, and both of them were fine with stopping.

I became a breastfeeding goddess among my birthing friends in the community. I was a go-to person for information and support, and on two occasions offered my own breasts and extra milk to help my friends' babies reintroduce themselves to the breast. Again, I never thought twice about helping when my friends brought their babies to me.

This most recent experience was the most difficult, and the one that I really feel has defined my relationship with breastfeeding. My newest baby was born with a short frenulum and a high upper palate. Translation: he had tongue tie!

Normally, this is a problem that can be caught within the first week of life and solved quickly, but it took two full months to resolve the issue in addition to weeks and weeks of pain and illness.

I am so grateful for my group of helpers who helped us to keep our breastfeeding relationship on track, and got us breastfeeding successfully. Our patience with the process really paid off. This experience of mothering through the breastfeeding relationship has had other pitfalls. I've also had mastitis, the "breast flu," with three of my children, in addition to the one with tongue tie, and I cry through the first week every single time without fail because I am so sensitive. I'm just such a mother.

I would have this no other way. Breastfeeding has made me the Mama that I am, and I'm proud to stand on the shoulders of Brown Mamas who have breastfed since the beginning of time.

Erica: A Breastfeeding Warrior

Erica has nursed one son heavily supplemented with formula, twins exclusively, a very sick child who underwent heart and stomach surgery before six months exclusively, and a *"run-of-the-mill"* baby who is still nursing. Here are some pictures of her nursing four out of her six children.

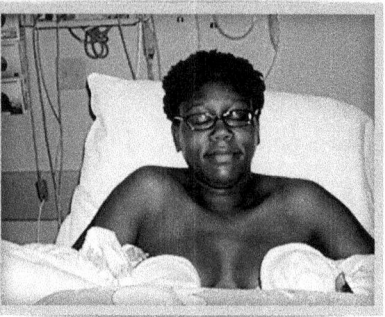

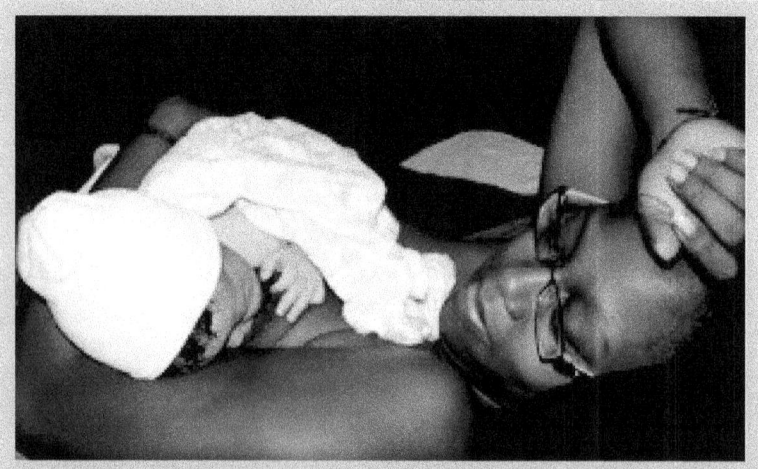

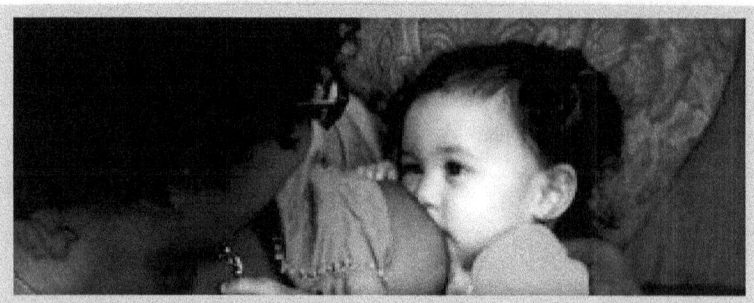

Chapter 5: Breastfeeding Warriors

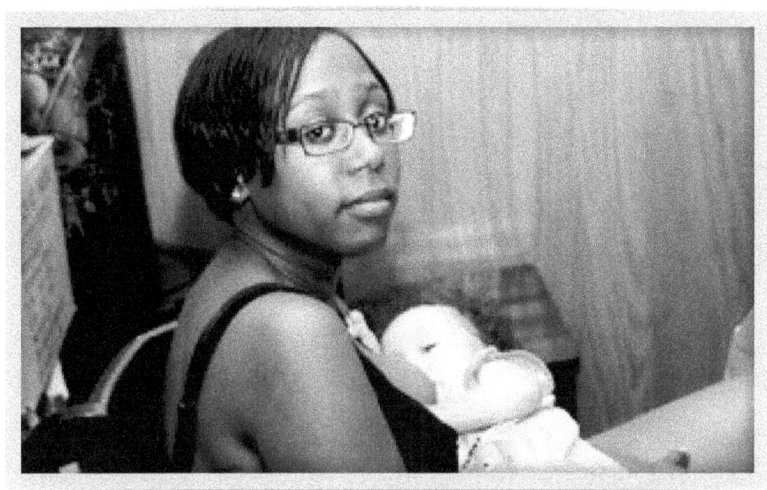

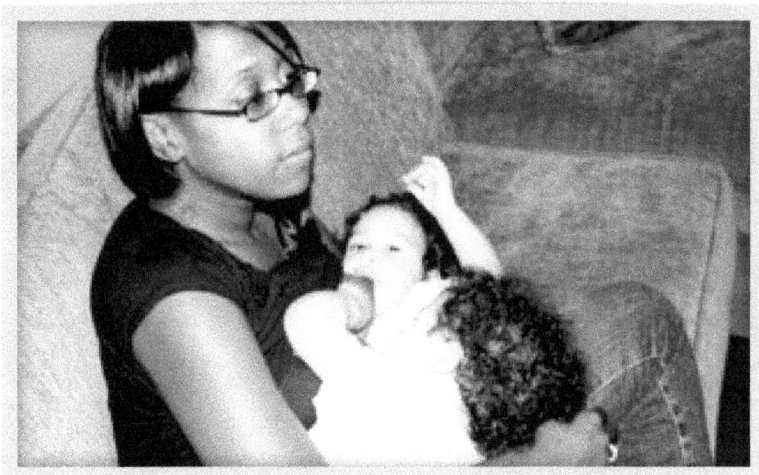

Breastfeeding for Other Mamas
by Natalie D. Preston-Washington

From: Preston-Washington, Natalie
Sent: Monday, October 25, 2010 12:21 PM
Subject: Resources to donate breast milk

Good day, all.
I write seeking your referrals on organizations or new moms who want to nurse their babies, but can't. I have a plethora of frozen milk that I began storing since late June. I honestly have more milk than my son can consume, and our freezer has little room for food. LOL.

I queried and she did not know of any organizations who would accept the milk—understandably for health reasons. However, I discovered this group GetPumpedOnline.org. I will pursue them if I have to, but I really prefer not to travel to Orlando if I don't have to.

Obviously, I was screened for everything under the sun before giving birth. I am willing to do so again if it keeps my frozen milk from going to waste.

…—I am thinking broadly that maybe a cancer patient is a new mom and can't nurse? Can you explore within Moffitt?

…—Someone suggested the Humane Society. I hate to think of my milk going to the dogs (literally), but if puppies can use it then so be it. Can you ask?

Thanks in advance for your suggestions.

Unfortunately, most of the non-work resources fizzled out. However, my day job—aside from being a full-time mommy, wife, and daughter—is in a college of public health at a major research university. This is where I was introduced to two babies in need.

Donor Baby #1 was the son of a former student. I befriended the mom during her master's program. At the time of our sons' births, she was earning her PhD. Due to medical reasons, the mom was unable to carry children after the birth of her first son. Thankfully, she is resourceful and was able to have a healthy baby via a surrogate.

Because she is a public health advocate, the mom began taking supplements to produce milk and pumped leading up to her son's delivery. She was successful and did produce some milk, but not enough to satisfy her son's appetite on a daily basis. As a student of maternal and child health, she understood the importance of breast milk—regardless of the source.

We had our first play date when I was on maternity leave and Luke was around 4 months old. Our babies played and we talked mommy business. At the end of the date, I gave her a few bags of fresh milk to try.

She was so appreciative.

Her baby had issues with the amount of my dairy consumption that was expressed in my milk, but she still wanted it. And, she found a way to make it work by mixing my "magic" milk with hers or formula. Once I returned to work, she would stop by every

Thursday afternoon for 5-10 oz of fresh milk. The weekly deliveries and occasional stockpiles of frozen milk continued for about six months. When the milk sharing came to an end, she understood that my supply was decreasing and I needed to save the remainder for Luke.

The family of Donor Baby #2 were complete strangers to me. A student and lactation consultant at my college shared my query for babies in need with her network of consultants.

One responded. She knew of a family whose baby was in neonatal care and still in the hospital. I connected with the father. He was interested and eager, but his son was very, very ill. Ironically, his son was at the same hospital where Luke was born, but they only accepted milk from a bank. It would be several months before his son was stable enough to come home. So many months had passed that I had written the family off.

Then he reached out to me again. His son was home and they were still interested in receiving my milk.

It was Christmas time and the temps were cold by Florida standards. But, that did not prevent the family—father, wife, and son—from driving more than 40 miles one-way to meet a family they did not know. Our encounter was brief. The wife slowly came upstairs into our home, followed by her husband and son. They had a portable cooler with ice. It was obvious from the frail mom that she was sickly, too. The son was small for his age and was on oxygen. Despite the cold temps, he did not have on a cap. I offered one, but they declined. I explained that after the long absence, I had given some of the milk away and only had 50oz (10-5oz bags) to share with them. Just like Donor Baby #1, they were very appreciative of whatever we had to give.

After about 15 minutes of exchanging pleasantries, they left for the long ride back home. My husband and I were not sure how to interpret the visit. My reservations were erased about a month later when I reached out to the dad again via e-mail. His son loved my "magic" milk and they wanted more.

Regretfully, our connection materialized toward the end of my milk abundance, and I was not able to share more milk with them either. Some might think that Donor Baby #1 and #2 were the benefactors in this experience, but I too received a gift.

I was so blessed and privileged to know that my milk contributed to the well-being of two babies in need. Additionally, the experience illustrated what being a mommy is all about—providing for our children.

Neither family asked for medical records or blood tests. They trusted in the fact that if I (a Black woman) had milk to freely share with them (not Black), then surely my intentions must be genuine. It was all about the milk and providing for our babies. Period.

The Life Cycle of Breastfeeding
by Tshatiqua Farrar-Baddal

Lacking a reciprocal bond with my mom gave me the impetus to make sure my children would have full access to me. The first attempted assault on this set principle came from the attending nurse at the hospital I gave birth at. She tried to dissuade me from nursing my newborn. I went on to feed her three years from my breast.

This inspired me to find a less stressful means of giving birth with my next child, hence a water birth at a birthing center. This was a beautiful experience. I learned so much about the birthing process, and was even encouraged by the staff to breastfeed. I began to feel empowered in my body's ability to bear fruit and sustain life. Finding an independent midwife, and arranging at-home births for my next two sons, was a no-brainer. They all latched on immediately after birth and have all, excluding my newest born, received at least two years of breastfeeding.

There is no substitute for the bond which is formed between a mother and child during breastfeeding. The eye contact, the smiles, the occasional tug of war as they rapidly pick and choose between the breast that is letting down the most at the moment, and the clarity you witness in their awareness of being, are all magnified with this precious action.

Making the decision to experience birth in its most sacred form and feeding my newborn children what nature intended, goes hand-in-hand with seeking to maintain a healthy lifestyle, primarily organic, with being a vegetarian, eating a self-prepared diet, establishing and maintaining healthy relationships, transmuting useless habit patterns from daily activities, implementing useful habit patterns in their stead, and more.

We breastfeeding warriors know that negative stress is the enemy of milk production. Therefore, finding creative ways to maintain emotional equilibrium is imperative. We also have to be wary of the introduction of non-labeled GMOs in the food supply, and the harmful chemicals, including fluoride, arsenic, lead, etc., in the water supply—as what our children receive from our milk is what we consume.

We have to educate ourselves and make healthy/ier choices. Altering the quality of life on the planet, for the better, definitely begins with us.

Friendly Encouragement Chat
by Celeste Jackson

Celeste: July 8 at 8:42pm
Something is seriously wrong with me. I put a metal bowl in the microwave to soften the butter. Good thing I took it out when I saw sparks.

Kenyata: July 8 at 8:42pm
U just still have baby brain...I would do things like that all the time until Haile was about 6 months or so...then you start to find the balance again...I'm still not 100% back to normal yet though because I'm still nursing...14 months in and I said I would wean him by the time he was 16-18 months old...U R nursing too, right?

Celeste @Kenyata: July 8 at 9:27pm
I knew I could blame it on the baby! All that DHA stuff...just my brain cells going to him. We are definitely still nursing and planning to go till he self-weans! It's so awesome you are still going strong!

Chapter 5: Breastfeeding Warriors

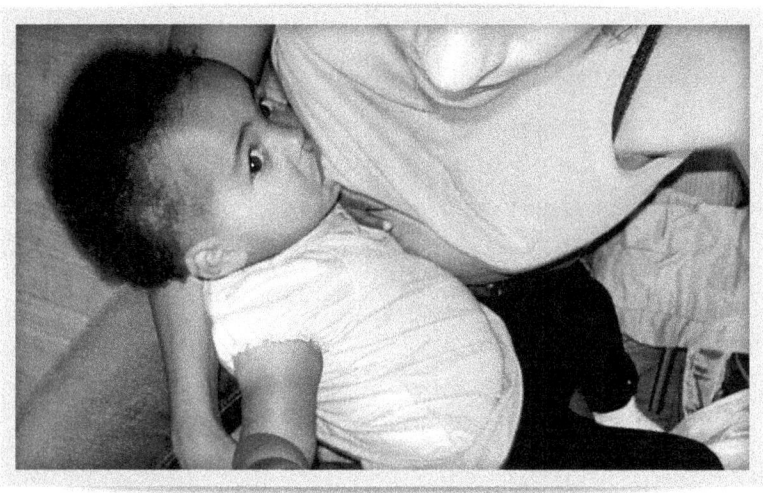

I Have Three Children, I'm a Breastfeeding PRO! Or at Least I Should Be, Right?!"
by Tiffany Chimaroke

Towards the end of 2006, I became a mother for the first time. I knew instinctively that I would breastfeed. I had heard my mother's stories of her breastfeeding my brother and me.

With my daughter, I was determined and very diligent about nursing her from the start. My birth experience with her was in a hospital, under neon lights, with the use of Pitocin and an epidural to keep me sedated and numbed enough to "push" her out.

My birth was vaginal, but in no way natural with all of the pain medications and artificial hormone enhancers to get my baby out. Three days later, as I was on the postpartum recovery floor, the lactation consultant finally came around to visit me in my room.

My breasts were engorged, and I was still unable to walk on my own as the epidural was still lingering in my body. The days leading up to my breasts becoming engorged, my mom and sister-in-law were consistently at my side trying to get my daughter to latch onto my breast. The nurses insisted on me giving her sugar water or formula until my milk came in. What little did I know at the time? The hospital staff were authoritative and pushy. I was vulnerable and new at this.

The hospital lactation consultant came in and corrected my positioning, ordered a manual hand pump for me, and then left the room. On day six, I was finally discharged from the hospital. I had also been given morphine during my labor, which made me delirious and wavering in and out of reality. My birth experience had been altered, and I had been released and sent home with eight cases of soy formula, Similac to be exact.

Upon getting back home, I had seven weeks to spend with my new little bundle before getting back to work, and there were things I needed to learn to do. I needed to learn how to get my baby to latch onto my breast correctly, how to introduce a bottle to her, how to pump breast milk and store it, and how to use the formula that I was given. I was completely overwhelmed.

Looking back on the situation leading up to the birth, and knowing I had to recover before heading back to work, was all a mystery; it's almost a fog how I was able to pull it all off.

My mother played a huge part in my recovery, giving me teas, making my meals, caring for baby while I showered or found time to sleep. She showed me how to sterilize the bottles, how to get her on the bottle fast, and how to use the breast pump. I was diligent and determined, but without her, I probably would have given up at some point. Her support was crucial for me to get through those early postpartum weeks and that initial learning of how to breastfeed my baby.

At about three weeks postpartum, I developed cracked and blistered nipples, and ended up getting mastitis on one breast. It lasted up until the time I had to go back to work. I was sick, still heavily bleeding from the vaginal stress of labor and lack of rest. Now, I also had an infected breast. I was stressed out and still trying to get used to a new person I had to solely care for.

Mastitis was no joke. It took my body to a level of postpartum stress that I had never heard about nor read about in any of my pregnancy books. I took antibiotics for the mastitis. I could not nurse my baby while taking the antibiotics, so for two weeks, I turned to the cases of soy formula the hospital gave me.

During this time, I tried to get as much rest and relaxation as possible. I ate foods that would allow me to produce more milk and learned how to use my breast pump. For those two weeks, I pumped and dumped. Once the infection in my breast finally cleared up, I was back to pumping and storing milk. I had only two weeks to pump and store milk before rushing back to work.

Once I got back to work, I was adamant about pumping and found myself pumping in the women's bathroom on my 15-minute breaks with the main door locked. Luckily, there was a refrigerator at work where I could store my pumped milk until lunch, or until I could make it home after work to my baby girl. At every lunch break, which was an hour long, I would rush home to drop off pumped milk and to nurse my baby. I would then rush to eat lunch in the car on my way back to the office.

Eventually, I talked to my supervisor about letting me have an office space to pump. After six months, I was given my own office with a lockable door where I could pump in privacy. This was my routine for a year. When my baby turned 14 months old, she no longer was interested in breast milk, and weaned herself off my breasts. Once our breastfeeding bond ended, I felt sad about it because I really wanted to continue nursing.

2008: Round two. I found myself pregnant with baby bump number two! It was a blessing, and I knew again that this time I would breastfeed as long as my baby wanted. My birth experience this time around was much different than before.

February 3rd, 2009, I birthed naturally, vaginally, and without pain medications or hormone enhancers. I knew my body could birth without those crutches, and I was determined to do without them. When my second daughter was born, she latched on right away, was very alert, and had a vigorous suck. I knew breastfeeding was the only way for us: my baby knew it, and I knew it.

The day after she was born, I was back at home, and my midwife came to my house to check baby's latch. It was all good, correct by nature. I went through engorgement, but it only lasted two days this time around. I used my breast pump to keep the milk flowing

Chapter 5: Breastfeeding Warriors

constantly. I was also able to release the milk by getting into the shower and letting the warm water assist in its release.

The issues came up later, as I found out my baby was allergic to several different types of foods. However, after changing my diet and drinking tons of water and liquids, baby girl was happy, healthy, and still nursing.

I nursed my baby girl until she was 22 months old, at which time I weaned her off slowly by realizing she only wanted to nurse for comfort, and not necessarily for nutrition. This was my decision at that time, and I was happy to have bonded with her for nearly two years.

February 2012: Round three, it's a BOY! I really was ecstatic to see that the baby I felt was a boy my entire pregnancy was indeed a boy!

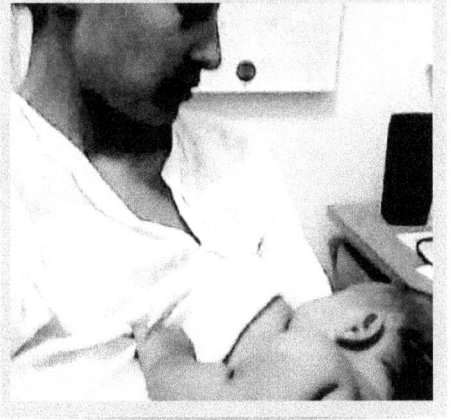

He latched on right away, but within days, his latch became poor, my nipples became inflamed and cracked, and my breasts were engorged.

I had no pump on hand this time around, but I had an abundance of local friends, family, and community resources that I could ask for help and support.

With all my experiences put together, I have learned a lot about the issues that can arise when breastfeeding. I know that getting the support I needed immediately each time helped me in meeting my breastfeeding goals.

Breastfeeding is something I am so proud of myself for doing, not only once, but all three times! No matter what the problems are, or have been, I would have it no other way.

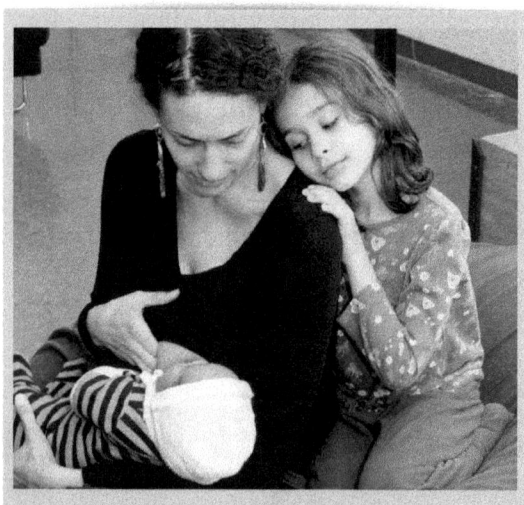

I am a Breastfeeding Warrior!

Chapter 5: Breastfeeding Warriors

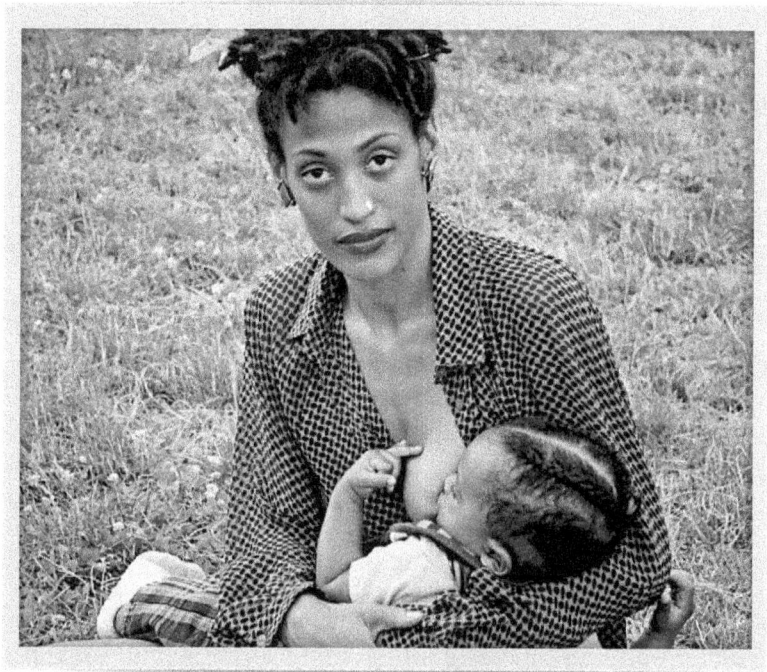

The Love Above
by Lyfe Silva

The journey to breastfeed Mason has been a rocky one. Initially, I had a hard time getting him to latch properly. On top of not having any immediate family members with any experience nursing, I was having a difficult time locating resources.

Luckily, I had a college friend who shared the same values, who was also pregnant at the same time, to turn to. She gave me some tips and encouragement. With assistance and love, I was able to begin exclusively breastfeeding Mason by month two.

Mason's return to this realm was a tumultuous one. With his father and I not being on good terms, we had to relocate to Virginia. Shortly upon my arrival in Virginia, I was determined to return to New York City. It was difficult because I had to start working and looking for apartments, so I made the tough decision to leave Mason down in VA with a relative for two months. This put a strain on my goal to breastfeed Mason exclusively, so for a few months his primary source of food was formula. I didn't do much research on formula, but I could tell the difference in Mason's demeanor. Formula was not the best option.

Once I got Mason back in New York, he was 11 months old. I began to research different alternatives to the formula, and my dear friend Anayah gave me a recipe for enriched almond milk and I was pleased. I gave Mason the almond milk, as well as my breast milk. Initially, I wasn't producing enough, so it was tough and frustrating for us both. But once we got back into a groove, my supply began to meet his demand.

Mason is now 21 months, and I am attempting to wean him, much to his displeasure. But it has been a long run, and I am ready to begin a new chapter.

Breastfeeding him healed me, and taught me about myself and the strength that I possess. It also linked us in our roller-coaster ride to stability. Should I have another child I will most certainly breastfeed; there's nothing more beautiful than looking down at your baby and seeing him suckling in joy and ecstasy.

Chapter 5: Breastfeeding Warriors

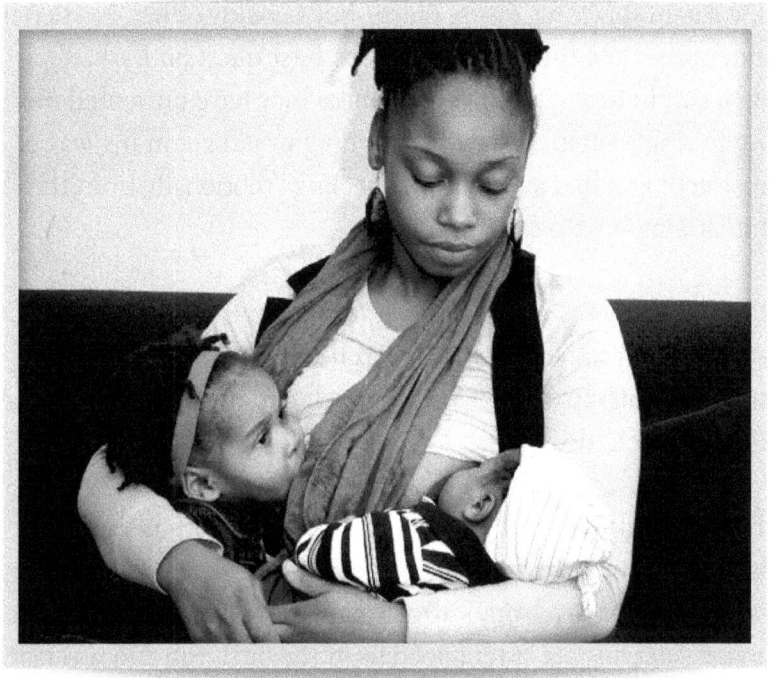

Tandem nursing
by Sona Smith

My breastfeeding journey began after an emergency c-section with my first daughter. It all happened so fast. One minute I was arriving at the hospital after laboring at home for a day. Then next minute I was being told my daughter's heart rate was rapidly dropping and she wasn't handling the contractions. Her heart rate was dropping and never recovering. Next thing you know, I was being put under: no time for a spinal. Strapped to the table, IV's going in, shaved, curtain going up, oxygen mask on, bright lights, no one there for me but me, and I was barely there. Count backwards from 10. 10, 9, 8, 7, 6, 5. . .

I woke up shivering, vision blurry, but I could see her. Nestled in daddy's arms in a fluffy white blanket. First question I asked was "when can I nurse her?" Circumstances may have prevented me from having a vaginal birth, but nothing would get in my way of breastfeeding. I had a rough time healing emotionally from the traumatizing birth I experienced.

Breastfeeding my baby girl always helped me get through the flashbacks and rough patches. It was healing to me. It helped restore the faith that I had lost in myself and my body to do what it was designed to do.

Fast forward two years, she's still nursing. My faith is stronger than ever. I give birth at home in the water. My beautiful baby boy was birthed into his daddy's arms and placed directly on my chest. Minutes later, his big sister joined us in the birth tub and was placed on my chest as well. She looked at him tenderly and they nursed together, and I cried as I had seen this exact scene in my dreams.

The month before my son was conceived, I had a dream. In my dream I gave birth in a setting that wasn't a hospital, but it also wasn't the apartment that I was living in at the time. I was surrounded by women, they were present but didn't bother me. They left me alone, but I felt supported. I had a sense that I was surrounded by a bubble.

In this dream, I gave birth to my child without any assistance, and he was immediately placed on my chest where my first daughter was laying and waiting to nurse with her new sibling. The baby immediately started to suckle, and then my toddler did as well. I awoke and at that moment. I knew if I ever had the chance, I wanted to give tandem nursing a go.

I never expected it would actually happen. Everyone told me I wouldn't make it nursing through pregnancy, that she would not like the taste of my milk and wean herself, or my supply would decrease or dry up altogether and she would wean herself, that it would be painful and too hard, etc. Absolutely none of that happened. She never showed a disinterest in my milk. I had an oversupply prior to getting pregnant, which caused me all types of discomfort, and in order to keep from getting clogged ducts, I pumped milk and donated it to two of my best friends for their nurslings.

When I got pregnant, my supply finally balanced out, and I no longer had to pump to avoid pain and drowning my child. I was sad about no longer being able to donate milk, but I knew I wanted a break in relying on the pump before the new baby would be born.

For the first time in my pregnancy my supply was JUST RIGHT for my baby girl. I also expected to get an opposing opinion from my health care provider about nursing while pregnant. However, when I told her I was still nursing, she was ecstatic and very supportive.

Our family experienced a difficult time during my 2nd trimester. My daughter and I had to adjust to a lot. Continuing to nurse helped me to ensure that she had something familiar in the midst of change. It also ensured that I took a moment or to each day to just BE and BE one with my child. This time got even more precious as I began to feel guilty about having a 2nd child so soon.

It helped me to feel as if I was easing her into life with a new sibling. And I believed as long as I continued to nurse her, she wouldn't have such a difficult time once the new baby arrived.

Things were going smoothly. Then in my 3rd trimester, I needed sleep. So I cut out nursing her to sleep and overnight nursing. It was a difficult transition for the both of us. However, I felt like I needed to begin to draw boundaries with her so that she would be prepared to have to wait and be patient so that I could nurse a newborn on demand.

As I got further into the 3rd trimester things got more difficult. I wasn't in pain and she wasn't showing an aversion. I just began to get touched out. I felt over stimulated, and nursing her for too long made me feel like I was going into a panic attack at any moment. I began to cut out a few sessions here, and there and by the time I was full term we were down to only nursing before bed and upon waking. All this time I had mature milk and my colostrum had not yet come in for the new baby.

A couple weeks before delivering I began to have prodromal labor and it really was taking a toll on me emotionally. The panicky feelings were more intense when I nursed. And I was having pre labor contractions every night for about 3-5 minutes apart for 2-4 hours. I just couldn't bring myself to nurse during that time. I had a conversation with her, and told her that she needed to take a break from mommy's milk and that the next time she could get milk was when the baby arrived. This helped her get excited for the arrival of a new baby. I did cave a few times and allow her to nurse, but overall we both did pretty good with holding out.

Chapter 5: Breastfeeding Warriors

A few days before I gave birth, I noticed that my colostrum was in, it was one of the times I gave in and she immediately got diarrhea. I figured it was because of the change in my milk. The day I went into labor I nursed her a few times to help me relax during some early labor contractions.

Once I gave birth to my baby boy, I asked her if she wanted to join us. The first thing she asked was, *"if she could have milk since the baby was here now."* I nursed them both and immediately begin crying because of the dream I had before.

We are now nearing the two-month mark of tandem nursing. It's difficult. I have a hard time nursing them together. I get the panicky feelings again due to being overstimulated. They have a very noticeable difference in latch, and suction rhythm and speed and it drives me bonkers. I manage this by only nursing them together if I absolutely have to. I also have continued to limit the frequency and length of her nursing session, because her latch is SO different from the newborn, and it bothers me. I can't really describe the feeling; it's not pain or discomfort, just different. It also is hard to nurse them both on demand and get anything done for myself or around the house.

I have toyed with the idea of encouraging her to wean sooner rather than later. But nursing her during this time has been such a blessing. It has helped her to connect with her brother. She takes so much pride in sharing mommy's milk with him. It ensures that I spend time with just me and her to help ward off feelings of jealousy. It helps me to manage her terrific-twos-toddler tantrums and meltdowns, which have increased since the baby arrived.

It also helps me to manage my oversupply and forceful let down without having to rely on the pump.

The newborn sometimes can't handle my flow, and nursing her first when I am really full helps to empty them a bit for him. Nursing her has given me so much peace as I was afraid that having another child so soon would force her to grow up too fast.

Tandem nursing has come with some challenges, but the benefits are too great for me to stop because of a few minor discomforts. I know it's worth it for the physical, mental, and emotional health of me and my little ones to allow weaning to come when she begins to show signs of readiness, and not because I have initiated the process forcefully.

Chapter 5: Breastfeeding Warriors

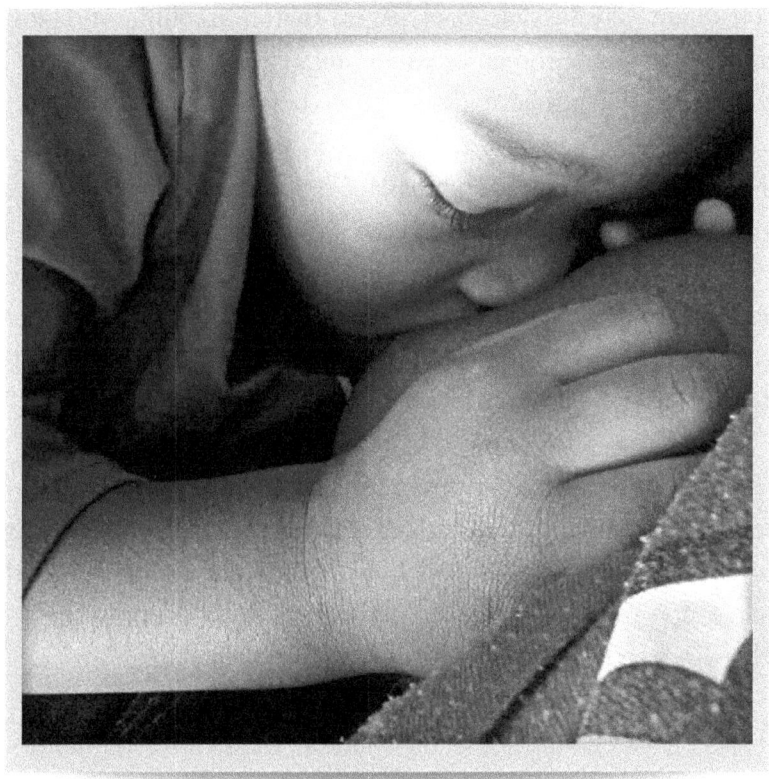

Reports Say Black Women Don't Breastfeed
by Darcel White

I am so happy to share with you this list of Black women who breastfeed! If you check the current data on Black women and breastfeeding, you'll most likely find reports saying that we do not breastfeed, we have the lowest rates, we only breastfeed for 3-6 months, etc. I would like to know where are the studies talking about the Black women that do breastfeed?

There are websites, Facebook pages, Twitter accounts, and blogs dedicated to Black women breastfeeding. I'm not saying the data is wrong. But I don't believe it's as dire as they claim it to be either.

I know that Black women breastfeed, and the evidence is on the website: *www.FreeToBreastfeed.com*. Some women chose to list how many children and for how long they breastfed. Some chose not to, and that's okay. It doesn't mean they didn't breastfeed for a certain amount of time. They simply chose not to include that information.

This list includes Black women from all walks of life. Mamas to one child, some with three and six children. Married mamas, single mamas. Some work, others stay home. Some nursed for six months, while others tandem nursed for years. Some used donor milk. Others induced lactation.

I also breastfed all three of my children. My first for 10 months, my second for 29 months, and my third 21 months and counting!

So let's get started...

• *Jatika and her cousin, Shanetra.*

• *@lawgurl*: Both children.

• *Dee:* 4 children; last one currently nursing over 2 years old

• *Melek:* Battled through biting issues and low supply from 9 months until he weaned at 12 months.

- *Dianthe:* Breastfeeding for 4 years. On 2nd baby and tandem nursed for a year.

- *Monique:* 13 months and counting! Her mom, cousins, and aunts also breastfed their children.

- *Angela:* Breastfed all four of her children.

- *Natasha:* 29 months and counting!

- *Sylvia:* Tandem nursed her 2.5 year old and 3.5 year old until she was 7 months pregnant. She weaned them at that time, and is now nursing her 3rd baby.

- *Tiffony:* Breastfed her two for 2.5 years each. Was breastfed by my mom until age 3.

- *Jamita:* Nursing for almost 6 years. 2 years w/Myles, 2.5 years w/Myla and currently nursing Mylex 14 months.

- *Tamika:* Breastfed for 27 months until she had to have oral surgery and was placed on medications for it.

- *Tiffany:* Breastfed both of her older children, and planning to breastfeed her newest arrival as well.

- *Kimberly:* Breastfed her first until he was 27 months, and currently nursing her 19 month old.

- *Kornika:* 10 months and counting!

❧ *Kimberley:* Induced lactation and breastfed two adopted daughters. Her oldest breastfed for 13 months but continued to receive breast milk until she was 28 months. Her youngest breastfed for 10 months, but continues to receive breast milk and she is 14 months. They both came off the breast when they were teething, milk not coming fast enough and constant biting. Side note: They both received donor milk PAID FOR by Medicaid.

❧ *Pamela:* Breastfeeding her son at 14 months. She plans to continue until he is 18 months.

❧ *Michelle:* Currently breastfeeding her 3-month-old.

❧ *Tiffany C.:* Breastfed her first till she was 14 months old; her second till she was 21 months old; and plans to breastfeed her new baby as long as she can!

❧ *Chalis:* Breastfed her first for almost a year (14 years ago) and is currently breastfeeding her 4 month old.

❧ *Kimberly D.:* Breastfed her first until she was 3 years, her second until he was 3 years, her third until she was 3 years, her fourth until she was 4 years, her fifth until he was 4.5 years, and is currently breastfeeding her 6th who is almost 6 months old.

❧ *Courtney:* Nursed her son until about age 25 months. Planning to let the baby still in the oven self wean.

❧ *Bianca:* Breastfed for 6 months.

Chapter 5: Breastfeeding Warriors

- *Rashanna:* Breastfed all three of hers; 8 months was the longest.

- *Sheril:* Breastfed five for a year each!

- *Kristal:* Not only was she a breastfeeding peer helper for the WIC office, she also nursed her FAB 5. One for 3 years...Breast ONLY!

- *Adiaha:* Breastfed two daughters. One for 2.5 years and the other up until one week before her third birthday.

- *Kanyla:* Happily breastfeeding for 7 months and plans to continue until her baby girl is ready to stop ☺

The Black Women Do Breastfeed blog and Facebook page are about making the community of Black breastfeeding moms visible. If you're on Twitter, follow along *@BlkWmnDoBF*.

Black Mothers Breastfeeding Association is a non-profit organization increasing awareness of the benefits of breastfeeding throughout the African-American community. Follow them on *Twitter @BMBFA*.

Blacktating features breastfeeding news and views from a mom of color. Elita's blog was talked about on TMZ!

Did you know that Michelle Obama breastfed her daughters? Erykah Badu has breastfed all of her children, and is seen breastfeeding her daughter in one of her music videos. There is also a great video called, *Black Women Breastfeeding: A Multi-Generational Story.*

As you can see, there are plenty of Black women breastfeeding. Thousands even! We have since the beginning of time, and will continue to do so.

When I put the call out for women to have their name included, I wasn't shocked by the response, but very happy and excited that so many of you responded. Thank you so much to all who shared with us!

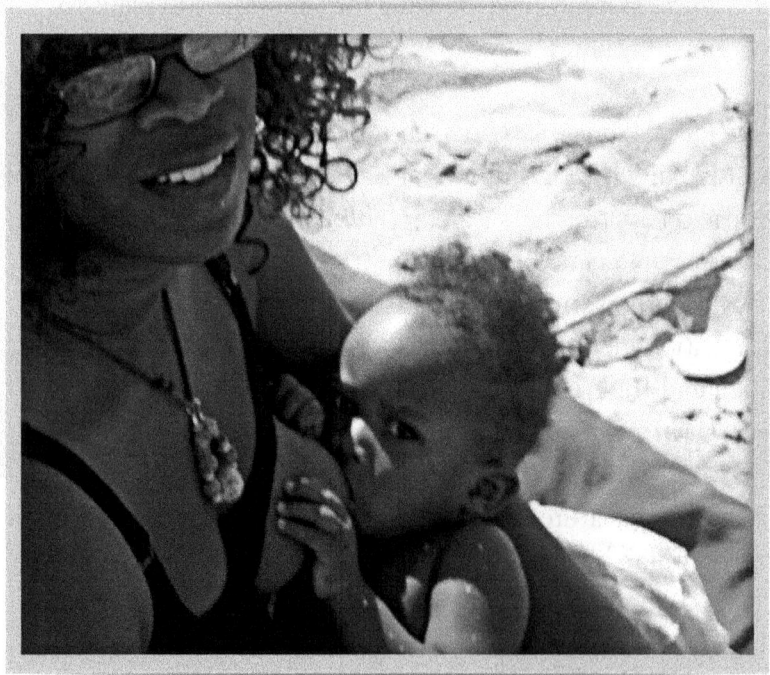

Chapter 6

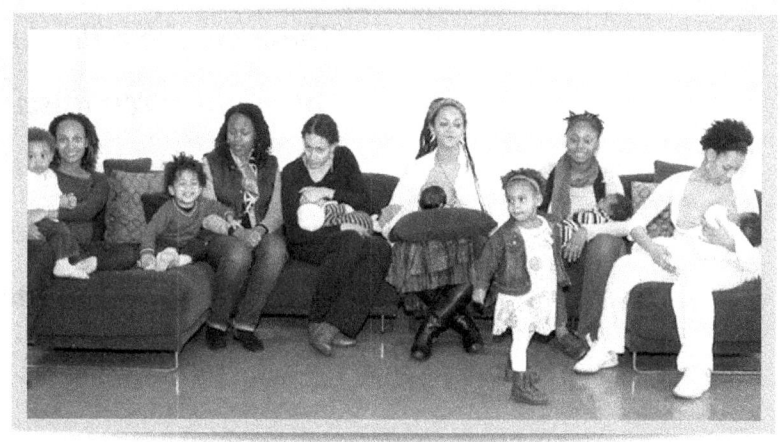

Coming to an End

It does not last forever. Though it may be frustrating, it is not everlasting. Though it may be a sweet nectar in itself, the breastfeeding relationship is still an ephemeral moment in the greater movement of life. These are the reflections of mothers reminiscing on the close of the breastfeeding chapter in their parenting lives.

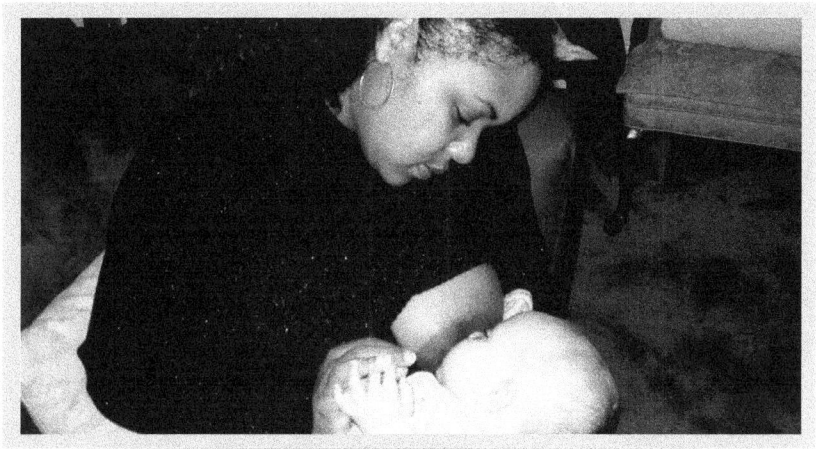

Weaning: Bye, Bye Hummies
by Yvette T. McDonnell

On Sunday May 29, 2011, I knew intuitively that it was time to wean my little one.

After fighting a urinary tract infection for over two years on and off since her birth, I knew deep within it was time to let my body heal, emotionally and physically. I woke up that cool morning and listened to my body. *"There was a shift in my energy. I needed to let go."* The first thing I let go was my shoulder length hair.

As soon as I washed my now inch long hair, I could feel the healing process begin. I felt and looked refreshed and renewed. I felt as if I had the strength to abruptly wean my beloved, despite the fact that she had already been night weaned. The next day was so special. I cherished each moment like a golden treasure. I thought to myself, *"She is unknowing about what is going to happen to her world and mine."*

I explained to my little one that evening, that when the sun came up the next day that she wouldn't have her hummies (what she called it) anymore. I explained to my little lovely that, *"Mommy had to take medicine that was not good for the baby, and if she drank hummy milk she would get a tummy ache."* My husband thought that was too much for our daughter and she wouldn't understand, but I knew she would.

Before my little one went to bed that night we took a family video of her nursing and saying, "bye, bye" to the hummies. I wanted there to be some sort of closing ritual and remembrance for her. My little darling nursed on camera, patted her hummies, and gave them a kiss good-bye.

That night before our little chickpea went to sleep, my husband and I lay on either side of our blessing, so close that we melted into one. I could feel the rhythm of our breath as we side nursed. I told my little one how honored I was to nurse her for so long (27 months), that I appreciated the special bond that we shared and that I had to trust my spirit that she needed a healthy mama. My husband and I lay there with her and we cried as she drifted off to sleep.

The next day my little darling woke up and wanted hummies. I explained to her that I wasn't feeling good, and mommy had to take medication that would make the baby sick. She cried, and cried, and cried. Her cry hit so deep within my soul, I cried along with her all day long. We cried together. I held her so close and rocked her for so long. I didn't interrupt our tears. We both needed to feel the sadness, we both needed to feel the separation; we needed to feel the moment.

Chapter 6: Coming to an End

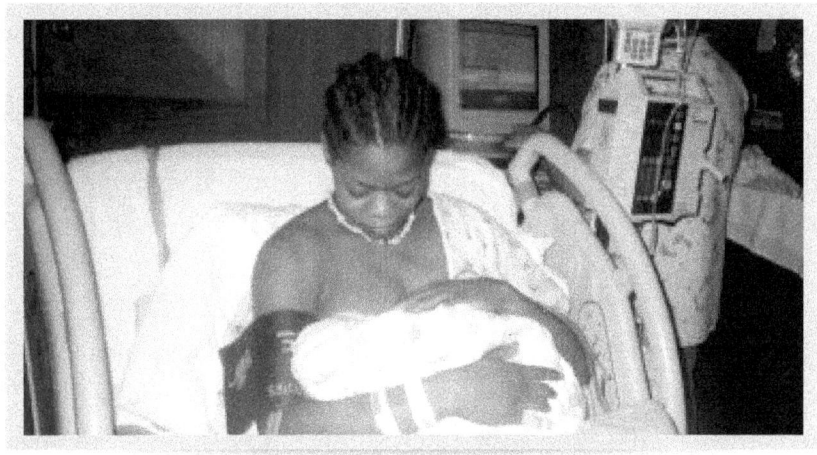

Hmph, Weaning
by Kay Harvey

Hmph,
I knew
This day would come
But didn't want to see it
I thought it would last longer
That sweet mommy/baby moment
My precious babe
Once so fragile and so small
So completely dependent on me
For nourishment, comfort, security and well-being
It's breaking my heart that this transition is beginning

My Ayo has begun self-led weaning
How I will miss these moments, suckling sweet
A pure liquid gold that comes only from me
This chapter of life is ceasing
My little boy is growing
Standing tall in his own being
But I know he will be fine
Healthy and strong
Because he had the very best start
As a breastfed baby

Weaning, for me this was the hardest part of breastfeeding. Simply because I wasn't ready. For me, it was completely unexpected. Ayo was around 8 months when it begun. He was becoming increasingly independent every day. He did not like to be immobile to nurse, Ayo wanted everything on the go (and 7 years later, still does), so I noticed that he began spending less and less time nursing.

Before I knew it, my milk supply was lessening. Then one day, it just stopped. He nursed that morning and afternoon, and that was it. He was around 10 months and was starting to walk well, and he wanted nothing more to do with nursing. I attempted several times for weeks, as I was in denial. I had planned to nurse at least for another 8 months. But Ayo wasn't having it.

So, even though I was heartbroken for those lost moments, I had to realize my baby was growing. So I continued to pump. But what was funny is that my son went from nursing to regular cups. He did not care at all for bottles. Breast milk did go in a sippy cup though to minimize waste.

It was our compromise.

Support Transcript
by Natalie D. Preston-Washington

-----Original Message-----
From: Natalie
Sent: Sunday, July 10, 2011 10:38 PM
Subject: All good things must come to an end

Friends,
Tonight (one day shy of Luke turning 13 months), I realized my breastfeeding days r over. And I am very sad. I had hoped to continue nursing at night, but busyness and some lingering health issues have forced my hand. I know I will miss it as much as Luke. On the positive side, I look forward to drinking freely while on vacay this wknd, wearing my pretty bras, and no more nursing pads!!!
Have a great week. Cheers, Natalie on her cellie

-----Original Message-----
From: Natalie
Sent: Monday, July 11, 2011 10:29 AM
To: [. . my Outpatient Lactation Consultant]
Subject: FW: All good things must come to an end

Good morning,
As of last week, I was producing 4-5 ounces a day. I missed a few nursings this weekend and did not pump--the pump is officially retired :-) How long will it take my milk to dry up? On a sad note, Luke woke at about 3 a.m. and wanted to nurse. Hubby tried to offer a bottle, but he wanted "magic" milk :-(I told him they were broken...
Cheers, Natalie

-----Original Message-----
From: [. . my Outpatient Lactation Consultant]
Sent: Monday, July 11, 2011 1:28 PM
To: Natalie
Subject: RE: All good things must come to an end

Hey Natalie,
You and Luke have been champion breastfeeders, so a big kudos to you! You are never broken, just moving on to the next exciting phase of parenthood. Still lots of ways to continue the wonderful bond you have established by choosing to breastfeed. Enjoy!

As to the question of how long you may have milk, you may still be able to express dribbles and drops up to six months after stopping, the usual time frame is about two months. Best way to minimize time is to avoid stimulation to your nipples (squeezing to see if some is still there and/or sexual stimulation).

I hope to see you and Luke at the breastfeeding support group meeting in August (5th). We will be celebrating World Breast Feeding Week with a cake! Have a great week.

[. . my Outpatient Lactation Consultant]

-----Original Message-----
Messages from other friends and coworkers who responded to my original message.

--Well, congrats Natalie! What wonderful lifelong benefits you have provided for Luke! I recently realized I'm done nursing as well. I'm sad too, but our nursing has been slowing down for about the last six-to-nine months anyway. I know I will always cherish my nursing memories and I'm sure you will too. Cheers! And enjoy that drink. You deserve it!

--You did an awesome job and gave Luke a good start.

--I'm sorry that you are disappointed, but I hope you enjoy the freedom!

--Wow, Natalie! You're good. I didn't realize you were STILL nursing. That's great! Be sure to share your success story with other new moms.

--You are funny. It is a special time, but as I said earlier, I was glad to be done. Now...stopping the "rocking the baby to sleep" habit is VERY hard for me. I feel like if I stop rocking her, I will never get to rock anyone to sleep again, ever. Urgh.

--Aw, hang in there mama. I know it's sad, but you'll get over it pretty quick. It's very freeing. :)

--My experience wasn't as positive, while I did like the closeness it provided between me and the girls, and how it forced me to slow down and invest the time, it was so darn painful. We could never get in the swing of it. So glad I attempted, but glad when it was over. Glad your experience was better, a closeness you and Luke will always have, breast-feeding or not. :-)

Free to Breastfeed: Voices of Black Mothers

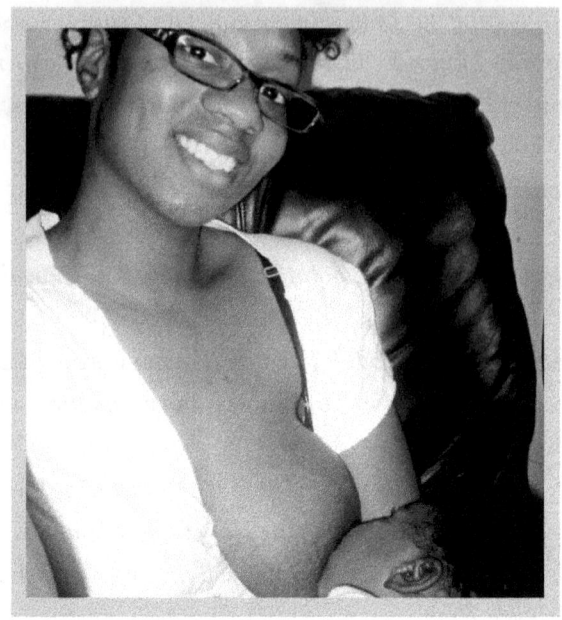

Power
by Ebon'Nae F. Piggee

I am a woman; I had all I needed to nurture my baby within.
A SUPER fuel
Not fully understood by science or men.
Don't confuse it with sin
It is pure, unalloyed
It is FREE, it is good.
WOW, my breast gave me Power; I AM a woman!

At the command of my baby, my body aligned instinctively.
I'd just lay him on my chest and as soon as his eyes met my breast, his whines turned into jest, and he'd frown a little less. All from the sustenance of my breast.

Chapter 6: Coming to an End

WOW, my breast gave me Power; I AM a woman!

I am a woman; I had all I needed to nurture my baby within.
But now, I was saying so long to my newly found friend;
I was just getting tuned-in to this power within.
Tears filled my eyes, when I thought about saying goodbye,
But it was no time to cry;
I was too thankful for the time.

WOW, my breast gave me Power; I AM a woman!

I am a woman; I had all I needed to nurture my baby within.
The capacity... I perceived that a woman could hold, sculptured my femininity and ripened my soul.
There were no looks or stares that could have deterred my goals;
No negative words or stories, I could have ever been told.
I did not look at the commitment as an inconvenience or load;
I just swam upstream and watched the logic unfold.
My baby was so secure and healthy. He exceeded all his milestones.
My mind and body felt great
I knew I had experienced all of this because of the liquid gold I was born to create.

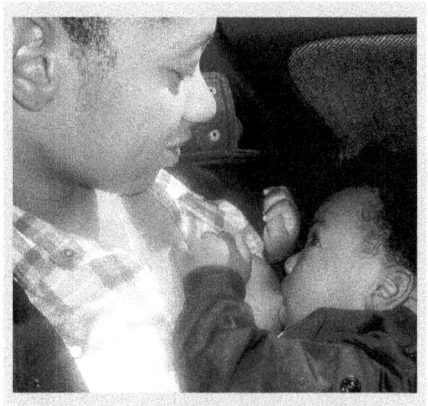

Wow, My breast gave me Power;
I AM a woman!

...My breast gave me POWER!

Useful Terms

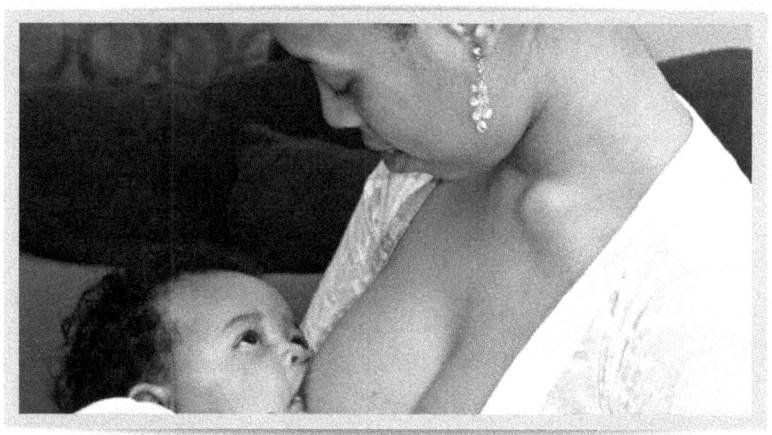

C

Cabbage leaves: a natural remedy for reducing milk supply including the treatment of engorgement, extreme cases of oversupply, and weaning. This remedy is NOT recommended for anyone allergic to sulfa and/or cabbage, and is not to be used on cracked or irritated skin.

Caesarean section (c-section): a surgical removal of baby and placenta through an incision made in the mother's uterus through the abdominal wall.

Clogged milk ducts (or plugged ducts): the back up of the flow of milk in a milk duct causing a small lump and/or tenderness.

Co-sleeping: practice in which babies sleep close to their parent(s), as opposed to in a separate room.

D

Diuretic: anything that causes an increase in the passing of urine (pee).

Doula: person who supports the expectant family through labor with comfort measures, encouragement, and basic lactation support. Postpartum doulas support the family after the birth and help build their confidence in caring for the newborn.

E

Epidural: anesthetic administered into the space around the spine to cause no feeling from the waist down.

Extended breastfeeding: breastfeeding beyond the first year, which is common in most parts of the world.

F

Fibroids: a noncancerous tumor located in the wall of the uterus.

Formula: manufactured breast-milk substitute or supplement.

Frenulum: the small fold connecting the floor of the mouth to the underside of the tongue.

G

Galactagogues: a food, drug, or herb that promotes and/or increases a mother's milk flow. Fenugreek, oatmeal, and nettles are all examples of galactagogues.

Gentian violet: an antifungal used to treat some types of fungus infections inside the mouth (thrush), and of the skin.

H

High upper palate: causes baby's palate to be too high for the mother's nipple to hit the roof of his mouth, resulting in the baby not knowing when to latch on and start suckling.

Homebirth: childbirth in a non-clinical setting, typically using natural methods, that takes place in a residence instead of a hospital or birth center.

I

Inverted nipples: the nipple, instead of pointing outward, is retracted into the breast. Some inverted nipples are pulled out by the act of baby breastfeeding.

L

Lactation consultant: a trained, professional health worker who specializes in human lactation and breastfeeding. Other health workers that assume knowledge in breastfeeding and support mothers in lactation are: lactation specialists, lactation educators, and peer counselors.

Due to the lack of trained lactation consultants, specialists, educators, and counselors in Black communities, we continue to have limited support in breastfeeding. If you have had experience with breastfeeding, consider becoming a peer counselor in your community.

La Leche League: an international organization dedicated to providing education, information, support, and encouragement to women who want to breastfeed. *www.llli.org.*

Let-down (or milk ejection reflex): when nursing a baby, the oxytocin causes a tingling sensation of milk rushing out of your breast. Let-downs are possible without even nursing (i.e., during sex or hearing a crying baby.)

M

Mastitis: a breast infection caused by milk stasis in the breast. Nursing-on-demand and continuous emptying of milk from the breast can prevent mastitis. Breastfeeding can continue with mastitis and can help to clear up the infection.

Midwife: a health care professional that offers care to childbearing women prenatally, during labor, birth, and the postpartum period.

Mocha Moms: a support group for stay-at-home mothers of color with information on childrearing and other family topics. www.*MochaMoms*.org

N

Natural birth: childbirth without any medical interventions which include labor induction, augmentation, and pain medication.

Nurse-in: a gathering of breastfeeding mothers and children in protest and activism for breastfeeding rights.

O

Oxytocin: hormone released by the pituitary gland that causes the breasts to release milk.

P

Poor latch: improper attachment to the areola and nipple, which is often the cause of pain during breastfeeding.

Postpartum depression or PPD: moderate-to-severe emotional disturbance, occurring after birth at a time of major life change and increased responsibilities in the care of a newborn.

Pump and dump: a phrase used to suggest the act of pumping breast milk and then disposing of it (dumping) for reasons that include medication a mother is on that is contraindicated for breastfeeding, drinking alcohol, and/or treatment for health issues that may affect the breastfeeding relationship. The pumping sustains the milk supply during the time baby is not physically able to nurse from the breast.

R

Reflux: stomach acid rising up into the esophagus.

S

Satiation (or satiation cues): demonstration by the breastfeeding baby to show they are full. Some cues include falling asleep, arms and legs extended, and arms straight at sides.

Supplemental Nursing System: a breastfeeding assistance kit used by moms and babies to help with supplementation. It can be used by adoptive mothers, premature babies, or moms and babies facing special challenges.

T

Tandem nursing: when two siblings (sometimes of different ages) nurse at the same time.

Thrush: yeast infection of the mucous membrane of the mouth and tongue. Mothers and babies can continue to breastfeed with thrush and while being treated.

Tongue-tied: when a baby has a tight or restrictive frenulum, which can impair the ability of the tongue to move properly to breastfeed effectively.

W

Wean: represents the passage of the breastfeeding relationship to another relationship. This occurs when a child transitions from breastfeeding to solely eating solid food for nourishment.

Wet nurse: a woman who is hired to nurse and sometimes care for another woman's child when the mother is unable to or chooses not to nurse her own child. Wet nurses were used throughout history, but they are very significant to Black American history. Black female slaves were readily used as wet nurses for their owners' children; often at the sacrifice of their own children.

Resources

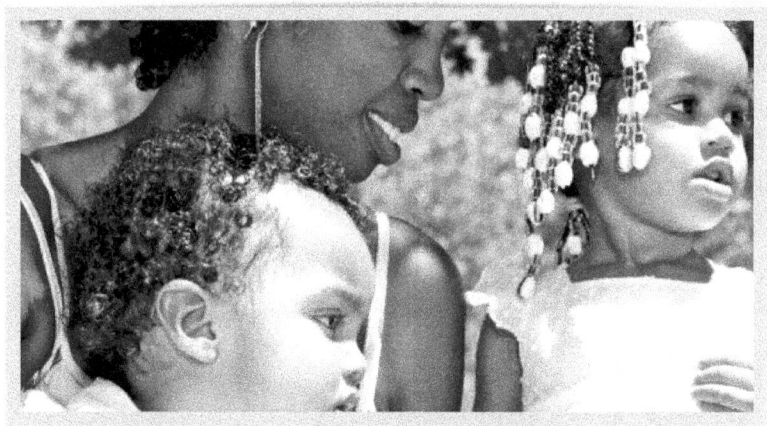

Books & Publications

Barber, Katherine, *The Definitive Guide to Nursing for African American Mothers*.

O'Neal, Mishawn Purnell, *Mommy's Milk & Me*.

O'Neal, Mishawn Purnell, *The Wonder of Mother's Milk*.

Pattrick, Chenniah, *This Milk Tastes Good! A Breastfeeding Nursery Rhyme*

U.S. Department of Health and Human Services

Your Guide to Breasteeding For African-American Women

Websites

Free to Breastfeed

FreeToBreastfeed.com

Blactating

Blactating.blogspot.com

Black Mothers' Breastfeeding Association

BlackMothersBreastfeeding.com

International Center for Traditional Childbearing

Ictcmidwives.org

Lactation Journey

LactationJourney.Blogspot.com

R.O.S.E. (Reaching Our Sisters Everywhere)

BreastfeedingRose.org

Office on Women's Health, It's Only Natural

womenshealth.gov/itsonlynatural/

Videos

Women's eNews: Black Maternal Health series

http://goo.gl/o4rL64

Sh*t People Say...to Breastfeeding Mothers by Anayah and Jeanine

http://goo.gl/374Vs4

Teach me How to Breastfeed by TaNefer Lumukanda

http://goo.gl/vGQCou

African American Breastfeeding Network, Breastfeeding Makes Strong Babies

http://goo.gl/0u26XZ

Contributors

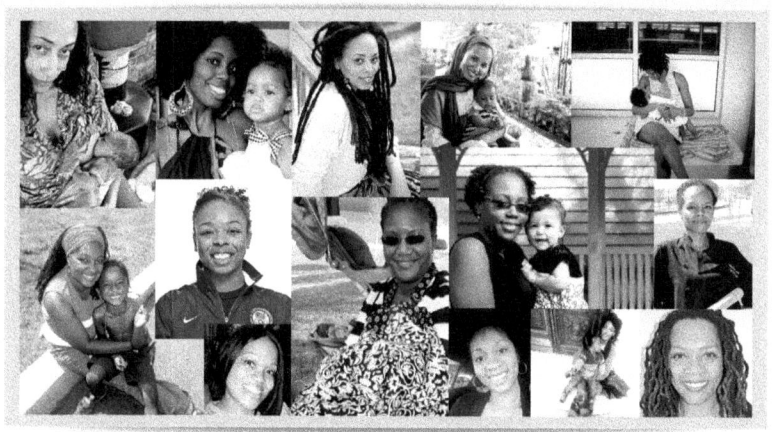

Contributors

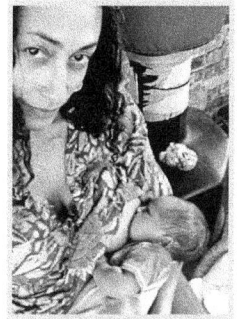

Tiffany Chimaroke is the mother of three children, has a degree in Urban Planning & Design, a graduate degree in Social Anthropology, and a Certificate in Sustainable Design. She has traveled extensively throughout Europe and the U.S., and is currently a Birth Doula & Reiki Practitioner studying Chinese Medicine with an emphasis in Holistic Health. She is passionate about Infant and Maternal Health policy, and enjoys gardening and making cloth diapers.

Kiara Diggs is a devoted and loving mother of two extraordinary children: Vivien, 3 and Sekou, 22 months. Kiara is blessed to be a stay-at-home mother, as well as an aspiring author, doula, and entrepreneur. She is a certified yoga teacher and holistic wellness practitioner.

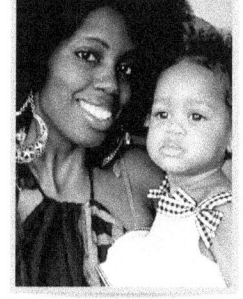

Kiara utilizes all of her spiritual teachings and experiences, cultural passion, and life experiences to help shape and mold her vision as a mother and woman. Kiara hopes to be a living example of greatness for her children through sharing her story. She hopes to inspire many mothers to take their own breastfeeding journeys. "You are not alone. There is a circle of women around you who have taken the walk. Embrace it!"

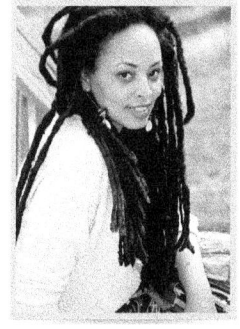

Tracy Eleazer is a doula, midwifery student, and natural birth activist. She is married and has given birth to six children (and stepmom to three), all natural. The last two were homebirths, one where a midwife assisted and the last one "unassisted" with just her, her husband, and children. She is a strong supporter of breastfeeding. She has over six years of breastfeeding experience, and is a firm believer that "breast is best."

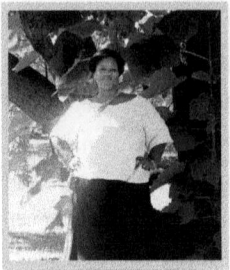

Tshatiqua Farrar-Baddal is an artist, songwriter, poet, aspiring author, and citizen of the world.

She is a wife and mother of four light-workers whom she homeschooled. She hopes to continue to channel beauty, kindness, and right action to all she encounters.

Parent, advocate, and emerging scholar, ***Stacey Gibson*** studied formally at DePaul University and informally by the folded back pages of Lorde, Kincaid, Morrison, Baldwin, Hurston, hooks, and others.

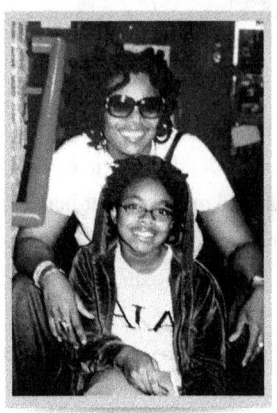

She has presented at national conferences including the N.A.M.E (National Association of Multicultural Education) conference, the White Privilege Conference, and The Unsettling Feminisms Un-Conference. Her current work on narratology, historicity, and responding to the oppressor's gaze leaves her wondering and wandering amongst the most damned and the most prolific. Ashe-O

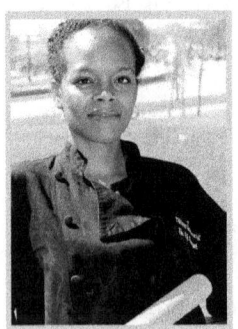

Chef Tiffany Joy Gorman has been writing poetry since she was 7 years old. After years in professional kitchens, she has turned to her first love, writing. An admirer of Nikki Giovanni, Gwendolyn Brooks, and Langston Hughes, Tiffany aims to project the same love and pride for her people in her unique voice.

This poet is the pastry chef of her own catering company, The Fif Element Catering, a wife, and a mother of one. Originally from San Francisco, she now resides in Chicago.

Contributors

Kay Harvey is a woman of drive. She is a mother, provider, organizer, and youth advocate, and has been working in the birth community for a little over two years. Kay is the owner/operator of Kindred Spirits Family Birth Partners (KindredBirth.com), a member of the International Center for Traditional Childbearing, and the Chicago Volunteer Doulas, and the director of the Doula & Parenting Program at the We Care Youth Center, which will be established in the Altgeld Gardens Neighborhood on the southeast side of Chicago. In her spare time, Kay loves to travel, cook, and do various outdoor activities.

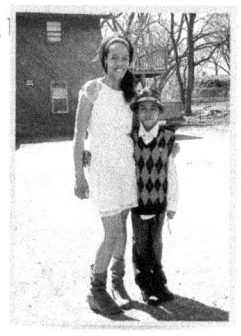

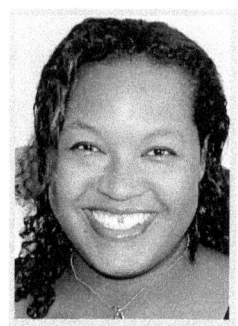

Sakinah Irizarry, 38, is a stay-at-home mom to Alejandro (3) and Maximo (1). She nursed each of her children for 18 months. Sakinah resides in New York.

Jackie Joice writes fiction, non-fiction, and poetry. Joice explores photography and loves to travel. Her new novel, *Kanika's Burdens,* was just recently published.

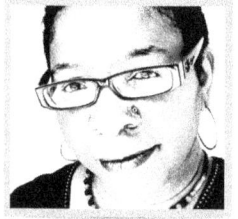

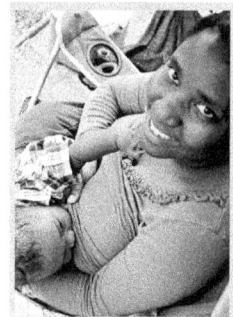

Celeste Johnson, is a 25-year-old stay-at-home mom. She has been married to her husband for almost three years, and is the mother to two breastfed babies. Celeste's son was born at home into the water, and she is thankful for her midwives and husband for all the help with her birth and breastfeeding support.

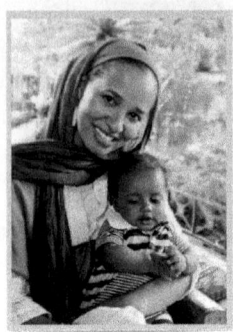

Ambata Kazi-Nance is a happily married full-time Muslim mother to one son, age two and a half. She is currently pursuing a Master's degree in English literature from the University of New Orleans.

After Ambata completes her degree she plans to obtain certification as a postpartum doula and a lactation consultant, which she became interested in while pregnant with her son.

Ambata moved to Addis Ababa, Ethiopia with her husband and son for a year following her son's birth and now is back home in New Orleans, LA with her family. She hopes to do more traveling as soon as possible, and is open to moving abroad again, especially to North Africa or the Emirates.

Ambata is an avid reader and aspiring fiction writer. She has written for *Azizah* magazine, and blogs occasionally at *GrowMama.com*, an online forum for Muslim mothers.

Patrice A. London is a Washington, DC native now residing in New Jersey.

Patrice is a wife, Christian unschooling mother of three lovely little ladies, a classically trained coloratura soprano, certified birth doula, placenta encapsulation specialist, and author of *Empowered to Birth Naturally: One Woman's Journey to Homebirth.*

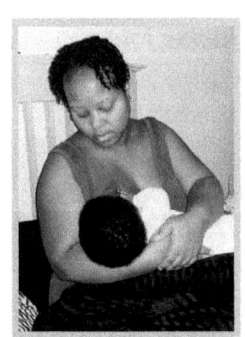

Patrice is also the owner of *Made by Love With Love,* making herbal products ranging from soap, salves, teas, and more.

Patrice is a graduate of Duke Ellington School of the Arts, and Bethune Cookman University holding a BA in Speech Communication.

Contributors

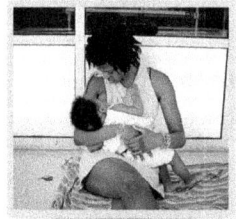

Jeanine Valrie Logan is a birth worker and activist, lactation education specialist, youth ally, homebirth mama, future midwife, and member of the International Center for Traditional Childbearing. She has worked for various organizations advocating for birth justice and safe motherhood. Jeanine is also a mama blogger *(ItsBetterAtHome.wordpress.com)*, and blogs regularly about breastfeeding, birth justice, and midwifery in the Black community. She lives in Chicago with her husband and daughter.

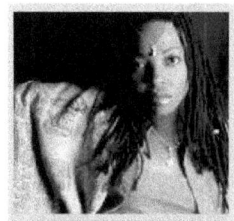

Mpho Venus Majozi is the gateway and spirit guardian of Jabari Khanya Majozi. Mpho is a seeker of ancient knowledge and a student of personal Ascension. She is a friend, healer, businesswoman, writer, and goddess of all things delicious. Jabari and Mpho live and love life in Johannesburg, South Africa.

Barbara Mhangami-Ruwende is from Zimbabwe. She worked in Germany before embarking on her undergraduate studies at the University of Glasgow, Scotland.

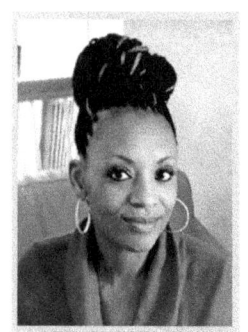

Barbara moved to the United States in 1997, where she attended the Johns Hopkins Bloomberg School of Public Health and Walden University.

She resides in Michigan with her husband and four daughters. She is passionate about raising her daughters, reading, writing, traveling, and running marathons.

She is currently working on a short-story collection and a novel. She blogs at *OnBarbsBooksWriting.blogspot.com*.

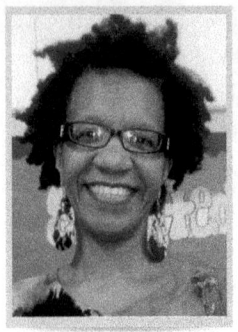

As a Women's Empowerment Specialist and founder of Choose To Evolve, **Kinyofu Mlimwengu** not only trains women on wholistic birth and parenting issues, but also on life and health issues.

She maintains The Self Reflection Blog *(EmpoweringWomensLives.com/selfreflection),* and creates conversations about choice, decision making, and self-actualization. She is also the proud mother of two future leaders.

Courtney Everette is a Chicago mama and wife living and loving in the southside. Her seven year marriage to Tre has borne two amazing children, Dru, age 4, and Kinlee, age 1. When she isn't scouting the city for fun kid activities, she's getting back into the hang of using her wildly overpriced degrees working in pediatric neuropsychology. Two high risk pregnancies, a surprise delivery in triage and 46 cumulative months of nursing later and she is still loving the journey of motherhood.

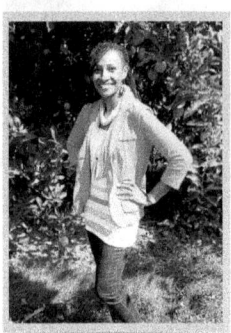

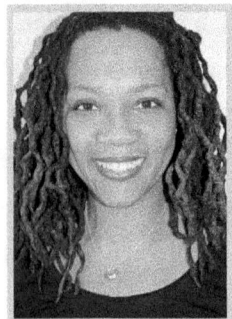

Kahlillah Dotson Mosley is an architect by trade, but mommy by choice. A graduate of Tufts University and Georgia Institute of Technology, she lives in Georgia with her husband and two children.

Kahlillah breastfed both children until they weaned themselves around 11 months. In addition to breastfeeding, Kahlillah babywears, purees baby food, and uses cloth diapers. She is a champion of breastfeeding among her friends encouraging them to nurse their children without shame or reservation whenever and wherever necessary.

Contributors

Erica McCabe is a mother to six children ranging in age from 13 years old to one. She is a birth and lactation advocate working with EMPOWERED Birth.

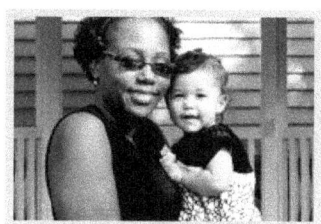

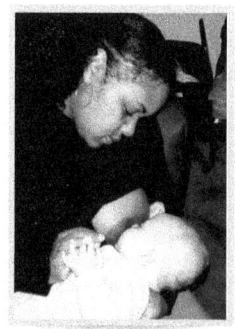

Yvette T. McDonnell is a professional belly dancer who left her career in Higher Education as a Diversity & Cultural Specialist, to dedicate her time to being a stay-at-home mom—"Domestic Goddess." Yvette and her husband Rob, homeschool their daughter, Anjali, and strive to live in harmony with the rhythms of nature. Anjali's experience breastfeeding for over two years of her life gave her a strong foundation and connection to her parents and the world around her. Anjali enjoys playing with her dolls and stuffed animals quietly, as she nurses and sings them to sleep. She also enjoys taking them for walks around the neighborhood in her homemade baby carrier. The family lives in and calls Maine home.

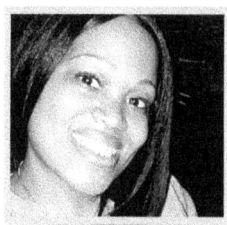

Evvett Pickens is a nurturing mother to Isabella, loving wife to Marcell, and awesome photographer at Evvett Marcell Photography, LLC. Evvett is also a proud member of Zeta Phi Beta Sorority, Incorporated. Evett and her family reside in New Jersey.

Ebon'Nae Piggee resides in Dallas, Texas with her husband, Shadrick, and their four sons: Justin, Christian, Caleb, and Collin. Ebon'Nae is a writer and natural childbirth advocate/educator. She loves to encourage women; she receives weekly guidance/encouragement as a member of the Potters' House of Dallas. She enjoyed breastfeeding her sons and hopes her experience will inspire other mothers to breastfeed—especially African-American mothers.

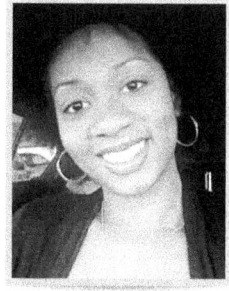

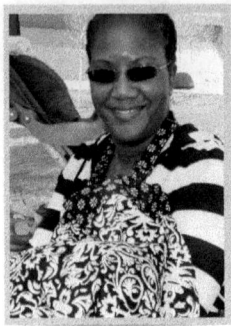

Natalie D. Preston-Washington is a certified lactation advocate, and provides support and advice to breastfeeding moms in her circle and beyond. On June 11, 2010, Luke Preston Washington was born to this mature, natural brown sistah. Knowing she wanted to breastfeed from the beginning, and thanks to an abundant flow, Natalie breastfed for an entire year (exclusively for six months) as well as being able to share her milk with two other babies. Her amazing breastfeeding experience has spawned her desire to become a certified lactation consultant.

Lyfe Silva is a mother, lover, healer, and artist. Hailing from Hampton, VA, Lyfe made the decison to move to NYC to nurture and grow as an artist. Born Aisha Silva, Lyfe made the change shortly after giving birth to Mason, who gave her new lyfe. Embarking on this journey of single motherhood, growing and nuturing creatively, Lyfe is presently in Brooklyn, NY studying biology. Lyfe aspires to be a holistic health practitioner and heal communities physically, mentally, and spiritually.

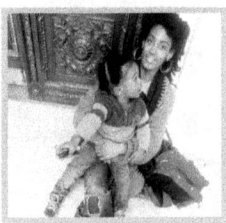

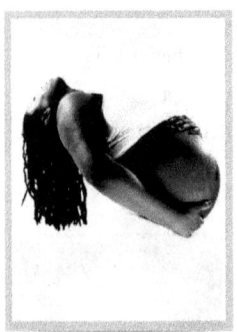

Sona Smith, Chicago, IL is mother to the Universe. Her children are affectionately named, "Sol," "Moonbeam," and "Starchild," and are her inspiration for living, loving, and growing. She is a doula, breast-feeding peer counselor, life-schooling mom, and non- profit professional with experience in youth development and public health. She is an aspiring children's author and plans to develop creative programming and products that support families to be more hands on, interactive, and engaging within their homes and in and with the communities around them to promote health, wellness, transformative learning, and enriching experiences for everyone. She is honored to be a part of this project and hopes that this book opens the door for more Black and Brown mothers to share their stories of pregnancy, birth, breastfeeding, and motherhood for preservation of the art of storytelling and to inspire mothers NOW and for generations to come. Sona can be found blogging at *www.BeautifulSol.com*.

Monica "NahZia" Utsey is a wife, homeschool mom of two vibrant boys, a freelance writer and part-time teacher with the Boys & Girls Club of America.

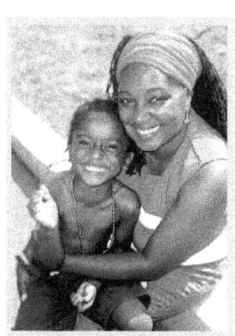

She is the co-founder of the Sankofa Homeschool Community, a support collective for homeschoolers of color in the Maryland, DC, and Virginia area, and President of the Southern DC Chapter of Mocha Moms, Inc. *(SouthernDCmochaMoms.org)* for the past 10 years.

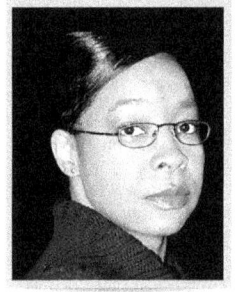

Tangela Walker-Craft is married to Ernest Craft, III. Married for over 19 years, they have one child together, Emari (age 9). She has a Bachelors Degree in English with an emphasis on Creative Writing from the University of South Florida, and currently holds a professional teaching certificate for Language Arts. Tangela is the Owner and President of Simply Necessary, Inc. which markets and distributes the GoPillow! *(www.SimplyNecessary.com/go_pillow.htm)* In addition, Tangela writes the Tampa Bay/Lakeland Parenting Examiner page for *Examiner.com*. Tangela and her family are all natives of Lakeland, Florida.

Darcel White is a mama to three. She is a blogger *(TheMahoganyWay.com)*, a natural parent, and an unschooler. Aspiring to be a birthworker, Darcel has always loved the 3 Bs—babies, birth, and breastfeeding. In her words, "I will cherish the breastfeeding relationship I've had with my children over the years."

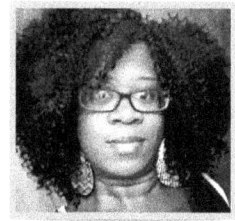

Forward and Cover Moms Contributors

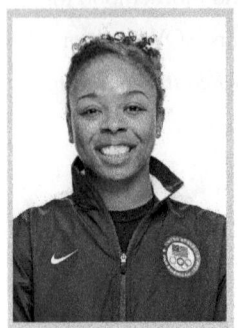

Angie Forsett is a mother, wife, and all-star-athlete. She was a 3 time All-American in volleyball at the University of California-Berkeley and joined the National Team in 2008. She played 3 professional seasons in Puerto Rico and 1 in Vienna, Australia. While training for the Olympics in 2012, she became pregnant with her now son Judah. She's married to professional football player Justin Forsett, they met while at Berkeley and they will celebrate 4 wonderful years this summer. Also, she earned a bachelor's degree in history from the University of California-Berkeley.

Yoli Maya Yeh is mother to Rhodes, a Yoga Therapist, Educator and Birth Doula in Chicago, IL. Through innovative education programs, Yoli supports social-emotional and mind-body learning through yoga, storytelling and play!

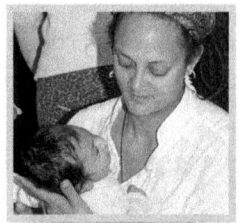

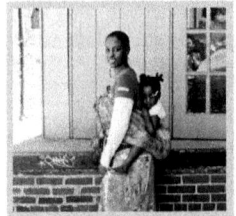

Nilajah Brown has had the honor of serving pregnant families for over 20 years. She brings a wealth of traditional birthing wisdom from African, Caribbean and Native American cultures. She is a professionally trained and certified mother, pregnancy yoga teacher, childbirth educator, midwife assistant, doula, doula trainer, reiki practitioner, and breastfeeding counselor. Reclaiming pregnancy/childbirth as a sacred rite of passage is her life's work and passion.

Dee LaCore is a student mom with plans to become a librarian in the near future. She loves knitting, gardening, and knitting in the garden. She lives at the beach with her husband and four children.

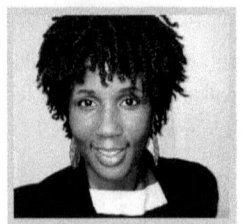

Contributors

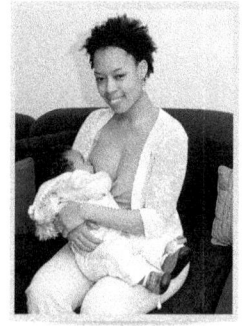

Zalita Zoe Neely is a first time mother who has successfully breastfed her son for 2+ years without the supplement of infant formula or bottles. She is an advocate for instinctive/natural/attachment/evolutionary parenting and takes a gentle approach to child discipline. She has a bachelor's degree in International Business/Finance and is currently an M.B.A. candidate for graduation. In addition to her foundational business background, she is experienced in childhood development. She takes her role in nation building very seriously and uses her opportunity as a mother to contribute to a more nurturing, compassionate, peaceful and loving world byway of instilling these values in her son. She uses breastfeeding as a way to support her son spiritually, emotionally, and physically in an effort to develop a well-rounded human being who would use his secure place in the world to make a positive impact globally.

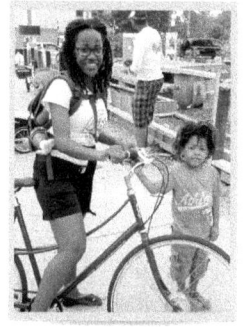

Latrice "Elle" Williams has spent many years working in the not-for-profit sector and is active in the burgeoning urban agriculture movement in Chicago. She is considered one of the city's young leaders in sustainability and has spoken on many panels and participated in conferences dedicated to climate action, adaptation and mitigation. She uses a wide lens to identify the various ways communities can sustain themselves with food choices being primary. To Latrice, breastfeeding is the single most sustainable choice a mother can make for the physical and economic health of her family. Latrice is a writer, breastfeeding peer counselor, women's healing circle facilitator, jewelry designer, garden manager, cultivation instructor and charter member of Bronzeville Bikes. She has been dubbed the Queen of Green by her project director from the Bronzeville Cookin' community development initiative.

www.ingramcontent.com/pod-product-compliance
Lightning Source LLC
Chambersburg PA
CBHW071717090426
42738CB00009B/1802